Enough is Enough!

Here's to your new Life!

Daniel H. Brin

Enough is Enough!

The *Cure* for Overweight and Obesity

David A. Rives

First Edition © 2021 by Moon River Publishing

All rights reserved. No part of this book may be reproduced or transmitted in any form or by any means, electronic or mechanical, including photocopying, recording, or by any information storage and retrieval system, without the written permission of the publisher, except where permitted by law.

Moon River Publishing
812 Natchez Avenue
Liberty, MO 64068
(800) 522-7735
Email: davidrives@hotmail.com
Website: MoonRiverPublishing.com

ISBN: 978-1-878143-19-8

If Nothing Changes,
Nothing Changes

> *Zen Bumper Sticker*

Preface 1

For People with Special Health Needs

As it says in the subtitle: this book was written to help otherwise-healthy people cure themselves of overweight and obesity.

As it happens, one way of doing that involves getting certain foods out of your life by eating certain other foods "without limit."

Obviously, if you're **not** one of those "otherwise-healthy" people—if you have heart disease, diabetes, etc.—then you really **shouldn't** eat anything "without limit."

So, when you come to the parts of the book that tell you to do so, do us a favor and ignore those parts, and just keep eating what and when your health professional tells you to eat.

Thanks.

Preface 2

Why This Book?

In this book's predecessors—*Walk Yourself Thin* and *Walk Yourself Fit*—we told you that you never had to change a thing about the way you eat, to get as fit and as trim as you'd like; that as long as you walked off every calorie you ate—and then some—you **would get fitter** and **would lose bodysize** (formerly known as "weight.")

Which is true.

So, why **this** book, that does talk about changing the way you eat?

Because even though walking **is** the only thing you'd ever need, to get as fit and as trim as you'd like, the fact is:

You can't always walk!

That's right: sooner or later, you're going to run into a day that's too hot, too cold, too windy, too rainy, too snowy, etc., to walk, which means you won't be building any muscle and won't be burning off any calories, which means you won't be getting any fitter and won't be getting any trimmer.

And even if you walk **inside**, on a treadmill or at a mall, there will always come a day when you're too "busy" to walk, or too sore.

However, even though you can't always walk, the fact is:

You CAN always change the way you eat!

That's right: no amount of heat, cold, wind, rain, snow, soreness, busy schedule, etc., can keep you from doing that.

So, that's "why this book:" because our job is to help you get fit and lose bodysize, and if you can't do it one way—by walking—then you're going to have to do it the other: by changing the way you eat!

Which is exactly what we'll be helping you do here—in the easiest, most fun way possible.

Preface 3

If there's one concept that's stood the test of time, it's this one:

Knowledge is Power

—the fact that the more you **know** about something, the more **power** you'll have over it.

Thus, the more our ancestors knew about where animals would be and when, or where fruits and nuts would be ripening and when, the greater their power to harvest those plants and animals when the time was right, and, by doing so, keep themselves alive, which, of course, is the highest "power" of all.

Yes, "knowledge" is and always will be "power."

And just because so many people nowadays are trying to convince you that the **opposite** is true, that **ignorance** is power—or, as George Orwell put it in his nightmare-world classic, *1984*: "Ignorance is **Strength**"—that the **less** you know about something, the **more** likely you'll be to make the right decision about it(?!)—that doesn't change anything:

Knowledge is Power

and always will be: the more you know about the world around you—and especially that part of the world we call Your Life—the more power you'll have over it; the better able you'll be to exert some control over it, so you're not being victimized **all** the time by those who seem to have "no problem" controlling it **for** you—food companies, tobacco companies, booze companies, etc.—to **their** unending **gain** and **your** unending **loss**, no matter how much short-term "joy" their products might bring you.

So, that's what we'll be doing here: giving you all the knowledge you'll need, to take control of your life back from those "champing at the bit" every day to control it **for** you.

Naturally, those companies won't be all that happy that that's what we're doing here. In the case of food companies, they need you eating **all** the time, not just **some** of the time, the way normal eaters eat. Which is why they lace their products with one of the most addictive substances known to man—sugar—and then just sit back and watch you eat yourself to death, while they laugh all the way to the bank, and their Mercedes-Benz dealer, and their Gulfstream dealer, etc.

If you're OK with that—OK with being little more than a "crash-test dummy" for those billionaires, slamming into their "sugar wall" over and over and over again every day—then there's little we can do for you.

However, if you ever **stop** being OK with that—with being treated like the lab animal they need you to be—and you'd like to take your life **back** from them, then all we can once again say is: "Welcome aboard!"

Table of Contents

Chapter	Title	Page
1	"It's Unreal!"	1
2	"Gotta Have It!"	22
3	The Cherry on Top	36
4	"Hard-hat Area"	43
5	Normal Eater	47
6	By Design	50
7	Scary Movie No. 53	53
8	The Greatest Gift	57
9	Annie	59
10	Bobby and Dale	64
11	Scrubbing Bubbles	68
12	Perry Como	72
13	"It's Coming!"	74
14	Dead-end Street	81
15	"Play Ball!"	85
16	Crime of the Century	88
17	Night and Day	94
18	"Cheers!"	96
19	A Waste of Time	98
20	The Non-diet Diet	102
21	Pants on Fire!	104
22	Before We Start Walking	109
23	Walking	111
24	The Value of Walking	112
25	Lipo	115
26	The Greatest Feeling	118
27	The Golden Itch	119
28	"Just do it!"	121
29	"That's a Wrap!"	123
	The Log	125
	Appendix	138
	Glossary	142

1

"It's Unreal!"

As we've said, everywhere we can:

People who set goals, then work toward them, are invariably more successful than those who don't

—no matter what you're using to measure that success: money in the bank; living a longer, healthier life; leaving the world a better place than you found it; etc.

So, since they **are** so important, this might be a good time to take a minute or two to let you in on this **program's** goals—the main one being:

Getting unnecessary quantities of food in general —and of certain foods in particular— out of your life,

the same way they're out of the life of every normal eater on this planet; basically, to "cure" you of those quantities and types of foods, the same way we cured ourselves of them a few years back; the same way, if we were addressing a group of smokers, we'd be trying to "cure" them of cigarettes, and the same for drinkers and booze.

And how will we be doing that; how will we be getting unnecessary quantities of food in general, and of certain foods in particular, out of your life?

Of course: by getting rid of the thing that's keeping them **in** your life: **phony hunger pangs**; and, if you're more than a few pounds oversized, then they're **all** phony.

How do we know?

Well, how real could they be—that is, how could they be signaling a **real** need for food, your **body's** need for food—when that body already has weeks'-, months'-, or, in some cases, even years'-worth of food in storage?

Answer: they couldn't.

Then why do they feel so real?

Because the thing that's creating them for you, to satisfy its own agenda—which has **absolutely nothing to do with a PHYSICAL need for food, your BODY's need for food**—that thing knows that that way you'll always satisfy them.

Why?

Because that's what we're hard-wired to do: hard-wired to interpret every hunger pang as our body telling us it needs food, so what could be more natural than to feed it?

Answer: nothing—if it really were our bodies calling out for food.

But, again, how could they be, when those bodies already have enough food in storage—around our waists, hips, thighs, etc.—to last weeks, months, or even years?

Answer: they couldn't.

So, the question is: if it's not your body calling out for food, what is, and why is it doing that?

And the answer to that goes to the very core of our being:

Obviously, every one of us is born with automatic physical mechanisms for keeping us alive. I mean, when you cut your finger, you don't have to "think" your way to getting the blood to clot, a scab to form, white blood cells to rush to the area to fight off infection, dermal cells to creep out under the scab to form a new layer of skin, etc.

Oh no, all those things happen automatically, without any of us having to give them a second thought. And good thing they do, else none of us would have made it out of the first month of life, succumbing instead to massive blood loss or overwhelming infection the first time Mommy went "gonzo" with the nail clippers!

Obviously, that didn't happen. Which is why there's no doubt that every one of us is born with automatic physical mechanisms for keeping us alive.

But each of us is made up of **two** parts, aren't we: a physical **and** a mental? So, if we have automatic **physical** mechanisms for keeping us alive, shouldn't we also have at least one automatic **mental** mechanism for doing so?

And the answer is: Yes, we should, and yes, we do:

It's a little thing living inside our heads we call the Subconscious Mind, that makes us do everything we do (by the way, the reason we call it the **Sub**conscious Mind is that it does all its work "behind the scenes," as it were, so we're not really "conscious" of what it's doing; we just know that it is; the same way we're not "conscious" of the way our blood clots; we just know that it does.)

And how does this automatic mental mechanism keep us alive?

In a very simple way (and readers of *Walk Yourself Thin* and *Walk Yourself Fit* will already be familiar with this, though a quick review couldn't hurt):

Every day, two things happen:
- You do a lot of stuff
- You make it to the next day.

What your Subconscious Mind does is, it **connects** those two, thinking that the stuff you did was the **reason** you made it from one day to the next—not all that wacky an assumption to make, of course, since you did do both.

And since your Subconscious Mind's only job is to get you from Monday to Tuesday, and Tuesday to Wednesday, and so on, and since it looks for all the world like what you did on Monday was what **got** you to Tuesday, that would seem to make its job rather simple: just get you doing those same things all over again, no matter how absurd or destructive those things might actually have been (and please keep in mind: your Subconscious Mind makes no judgment about whether an action is "good" or "bad:" if you did it on Monday and made it to Tuesday, it thinks you **needed** to do it on Monday to make it to Tuesday, and it's going to **keep** making you do it till you tell it to stop!)

And how does your Subconscious Mind get you doing the same things over and over again, day after day?

Easy: by creating a hunger, a craving, to do those things that's all-but-impossible to resist. So you don't resist it. Instead you give in to it, thinking that, by doing so, you're doing the best thing for yourself you possibly could.

Except…you're not.

In fact, when it comes to abusive eating (or smoking or drinking), you're doing the **worst** thing for yourself you possibly could, as any number of life-expectancy charts will gladly tell you.

Doesn't matter: have a dozen chocolate chip cookies on Monday and make it to Tuesday and your Subconscious Mind will think those cookies were the **reason** you made it to Tuesday. And, since its only job is to get you to Wednesday, that would seem to make its job rather simple: just get you eating a dozen chocolate chip cookies all over again on Tuesday. Which it does: by creating a hunger, a craving, for those cookies that's impossible to resist.

And, when you have those cookies on Tuesday and make it to Wednesday, that "proves" to your Subconscious Mind that it was right: that you did need those cookies on Tuesday to make it to Wednesday, so it has "no problem" making you hungry for another dozen chocolate chip cookies on Wednesday, which it does by creating a hunger…well, this is where we came in.

So, there you have it: the cause of all the overweight and obesity in this country—and, increasingly, the world: your **brain** taking control of a part of your **body**—your stomach—to get you doing what **it** wants you to do, what it thinks you **need** to do, to survive.

In other words, acting very much like a **virus**, which functions by "taking over" a cell and then using that cell's machinery to do **its** bidding, rather than that of the cell it's taken over.

Which, of course, is the best news we could possibly get. Why?

Because that means that all we have to do is fix **that one thing**—that out-of-control Subconscious Mind—and our problem will be solved.

And how do we fix it?

Well, how did we "break" it?

Of course: by "feeding" it cookies and Pop-tarts on Monday, then making it to Tuesday, so that it had "no choice" but to make us hungry for cookies and Pop-tarts all over again on Tuesday.

The solution?

Of course: **stop** feeding it cookies and Pop-tarts on Monday.

"So that's it: just stop having that stuff on Monday and my Subconscious Mind will simply back off and leave me alone?"

Uh, no—that's not what's going to happen.

"Why not?"

Because your Subconscious Mind really does think those cookies and Pop-tarts were the reason you made it from Monday to Tuesday. Which means that, the minute you **stop** having those cookies and Pop-tarts, your Subconscious Mind will think you're **trying to kill yourself** and it **can't let that happen**!

And how does it **keep** that from happening?

In more ways than you can count (and anyone who's ever gone on a diet will be familiar with every one of these, though you may not have known where they came from):

1) The first thing your Subconscious Mind does, when it sees those cookies and Pop-tarts have stopped coming its way, is: it **doubles and triples the intensity of your hunger pangs**.

Why?

Because **it** knows that **you** know that all it would take, to make those pangs go away, would be a cookie or two. Which, when the pain becomes unbearable, is exactly what you give it, thereby letting it put a star on **its** forehead and another pound or two on **yours**!

2) And if you decide to "tough it out;" to not give it the cookies and Pop-tarts it's calling for?

Well, then it pulls out the next arrow in its quiver: cutting off the blood flow to the wakefulness center in your brain, thereby turning you into a "zombie," unable to stay awake, do a lick of work, etc.

And why does it do that?

Because **it** knows that **you** know that all it would take, to get you bright and perky again, would be a cookie or two. Which, more often than not, is what you wind up giving it.

3) And if you don't give it that cookie or two—if you say to yourself, "Well, I'll just let my body pull some cookies out of storage, and use **those** to get my energy back up"—what your Subconscious Mind does is, it says, "Oh yeah? Well, we'll see about that!" and promptly cuts off the flow of blood into and out of your **fat pads**, so that all those stored cookies might just as well be on Mars, for all the good they're going to do you!

And why does it do that?

Because **it** knows that **you** know that, if you can't use your **stored** cookies to get rid of the hunger pangs and the tiredness, then you're going to have to turn to the only place you can for those cookies: the outside world. Which, more often than not, you do.

And on and on it goes, with your Subconscious Mind doing everything in its power to get you eating again, and with you doing everything in your power to resist it.

In other words, what shapes up as nothing less than a **war**, between you and your Subconscious Mind!

Obviously, if **it** wins the war, your life will be filled with nonstop eating, nonstop size gain, nonstop health problems, etc., whereas, if **you** win the war, your life will be filled with normal eating, a return to normal size, lowered risk of getting an endless number of obesity-related diseases (diabetes, stroke, high blood pressure, arthritis, a number of cancers); etc.

That's it; that's your choice.

Obviously, we're here to help **you** win that war.

How?

Well mainly, by letting you know why you eat the way you do, then giving you the tools to stop eating that way, if you want.

Naturally, some of you will embrace this knowledge and run with it; will use it to take your life back from Sara Lee and Ronald McDonald and Tony the Tiger and the Pillsbury Doughboy and the Keebler Elves, and all the other cutesy-pie characters the food companies have come up with, to lull you into thinking that consuming their products is the most fun, harmless thing a human being could be doing with its life, the same way the R. J. Reynolds Tobacco Company came up with Joe Camel a few years back, to lull 10- and 12-year-olds into thinking that consuming **their** product was the most fun, harmless thing a **child** could be doing with its life—to which all we can say is: hop on down to your nearest stage 4 lung cancer center, with its row after row of "living corpses," and then let me know how many times the words "fun" and "harmless" come to mind!

Yes, some of you will embrace this knowledge and run with it.

Unfortunately, just as many of you will turn your **back** on this knowledge and run **from** it.

Why?

Because what we're talking about here involves making a change in your life, and if there's one thing we humans hate above all else, it's: change.

In fact, every time a list comes out, of the most stressful things a human being can go through, nearly all of them involve some sort of change:
- Going off to school
- Leaving school
- Getting a job
- Losing a job
- Getting married
- Getting divorced
- Moving house
- Losing a loved one.

No, the fact is, most people would rather die than change—or, as Thomas Jefferson put it, in America's Declaration of Independence: "…all experience hath shewn that mankind are more disposed to suffer, while evils are sufferable, than to right themselves by abolishing the forms to which they are accustomed."

In other words, most people would rather die than change—and do so with depressing regularity!

So, no: you don't want to change, because none of us does. Much easier to just keep having those pancakes day after day; that mountain of mashed potatoes-and-gravy; those 20 trips to the all-you-can-eat buffet tables; etc.

And yet, change we must, if we're ever going to move forward in this life, since we all know the definition of insanity: Doing things the way you've always done them, yet expecting different results.

Meaning that it would be nothing less than "insane" to think we could keep eating the way we've been eating and yet wind up turning ourselves into normal-sized normal eaters.

So, again: most people would rather die than change, and yet change we must, if we're ever going to get anywhere.

So, what does that tell us?

Well, if nothing else, it tells us we'd better make those changes as easy and painless as possible—ideally, something we call a "no-brainer," where, if you just follow a series of simple steps, you'll reach your goal, no matter what that goal might be.

Which, hopefully, is exactly what we've done here.

Of course, even though we might make **individual** changes as simple as possible, that still doesn't mean that **change**, **itself**, will be all that easy.

Why not?

Well, first of all, because, as we've just gone into, **you** don't want to change, because no one ever does.

But there's more to it than that: obviously,

• The **food companies** don't want you to change because they're making a fortune off you.

So, don't hold your breath waiting for them to slap a warning on their packages, like the ones you see on cigarette packs, letting you know that their products will basically kill you if you consume more than a tiny amount of them.

• Certain members of the **medical-pharmaceutical complex** don't want you to change because **they're** making a fortune off you—off the diseases you most likely never would have gotten, if you'd exercised your legs a little more, the last 10 or 20 years, and your fork a little less.

• The **government** doesn't want you to change, because those food companies and medical companies employ a lot of people, so the government doesn't have to, and they pay a lot of taxes, so the government can keep its doors open.

So don't hold your breath waiting for your government to **make** those food companies put warnings on their packages, because then they'd be "killing the goose that's been laying the golden eggs," and nobody does that if he can help it.

• Your **friends** don't want you to change because, more often than not, they're the same size you are, and anytime you start taking steps to **change** that size—for example, by changing the way you eat—it starts looking like you're trying to show them up, and friends just don't do that to friends. So, to "keep the peace," you keep stuffing your face with the best of them.

So, no: change is never easy. Which is why we've tried to make each step along the way as simple as possible.

So, that's what we'll be doing here: giving you a series of simple steps, to enable you to take yourself from the eating life you're currently living to the eating life you should have been living all along, and would have been living, if someone hadn't given you a different one, long before you were old enough or smart enough to know what they were doing to you; in other words, long before you were old enough or smart enough to stop them—unless you'd like to try making a living by getting a dollar for every five-year-old who stands up, after his mother has plunked down a stack of syrup-soaked pancakes in front of him, and says, "Excuse me, mother, but what you've just given me is not, in fact, 'food;' is, in fact, little more than a 'dessert,' which, like most desserts, will do nothing for me but make me fat, rot my teeth, clog my arteries, and get me addicted to it—and all while giving me not a nickel's-worth of nutrition in return.

"So, just this once—and possibly forever—I'm going to be taking a 'pass' on those pancakes, and having the breakfast normal eaters have: an egg, a piece of toast, and a glass of orange juice."

Yeah, right: you hold your breath waiting for **that** to happen!

Oh no: Mommy plunks down a stack of pancakes in front of five-year-old you, you're going to eat them!

Why?

Well, why wouldn't you: after all, Mommies are big, you're small; Mommies are smart, you're…well, not so much yet.

So, if Mommy is giving you those pancakes, she must know what she's doing, right?

I mean, like every Mommy, she only has your best interests at heart, so why would she give you something that would harm you?

Well, how much time have you got:

1) First of all, as we brought up in *Walk Yourself Thin* and *Walk Yourself Fit*: there are more than a few Mommies out there who know, to a dead certainty, that someone from the Starvation Patrol is camped outside their door, 24/7, just waiting to haul them off to Bad Mommy Prison at the first sign of an undernourished child. So, like it or not, you're going to get fed—a million times a day, if necessary.

And since Mommy knows you'll **never** turn down pancakes-and-maple syrup; or biscuits-and-gravy; or bowl after bowl of Lucky Charms or Cap'n Crunch—because she knows you'll never turn those down, that, in fact, is what you get. Which then proceed to do to you exactly what our little five-year-old said they would: make you fat, rot your teeth, clog your arteries, and get you addicted to them—and all without giving you so much as a nickel's-worth of nutrition in return.

So that's reason number one that Mommy gives you all that garbage: because she knows you'll eat it, so at least you'll **look** well-fed, even if you're not, which means she won't be getting hauled off to Bad Mommy Prison anytime soon.

But there's more:

2) The main reason your Mommy gives you those things is because that's what **her** Mommy gave **her**; and what **her** Mommy's Mommy gave **your** Mommy's Mommy—and so on and so on, until, I guess, you wind up back at Adam and Eve—or at least, the Great Depression!

And, again, since Mommies are "infallible" in a 5-year-old's eyes, then, if your Mommy's Mommy fed **your** Mommy pancakes, then that's what **your** Mommy's going to feed **you**—and do so without seeing the slightest thing wrong in it, even though it is, in fact, most likely the "**wrongest**" thing she could possibly be doing to you!

Oh no: if your Mommy's Mommy gave your Mommy pancakes, then why would your Mommy have a problem giving them to you?

Answer: she wouldn't. And doesn't.

Which is how things like pancakes, and fried pig fat, and cinnamon rolls, and biscuits-and-gravy, and hash browns, and apple pie, and Honey Bunches of Oats, and caramel macchiatos, and all their "cousins" became "acceptable fare" for the morning meal—when, in fact, those are the **last** things any human being should be eating.

The problem is: there was a time—and not that long ago—when there was, in fact, **nothing wrong** with having any or all of those things for breakfast.

Why not?

Because within minutes of finishing those pancakes, cinnamon rolls, gravy biscuits, etc., you'd be hitching your horse to a plow and walking behind it for the next 10 hours—burning up every calorie you just ate, as you "worked the 'north 40.'"

Which is fine, except: the only "north 40" most of us are "working" nowadays are the top 40 singles on Spotify!

And there's the problem; the answer to how this country became the fattest nation in the history of the world:

We stopped moving, but forgot to stop eating!

That's right: as long as we were doing something physical 10 hours a day, it didn't matter what we ate: those activities would burn off every calorie!

But we're **not** doing something physical 10 hours a day anymore, are we? In fact, from the looks of it, most of us aren't doing something physical 10 **minutes** a day—forget **hours**!—which, of course, hasn't stopped us from **eating** like we were!

So, again, the answer to how we got so fat:

We stopped moving, but forgot to stop eating!

The solution?

Obviously: either stop eating or start moving again. Or (could we be so lucky?): **both**.

We've pretty much taken care of the "moving" part of the equation, with the *Walk Yourself Thin* and *Walk Yourself Fit* programs (which we'll review and expand on, later in the book.)

So, all that's left is the "stop eating" part (and please understand: when we say "stop eating," all we mean is: stop eating more calories than you'll be using up in the course of a day—especially calories in the form of things like cookies and candy and cake and ice cream.)

So, that's what this book is all about: giving you the tools to stop eating excessive quantities of food in general—and of certain foods in particular—and thereby taking you to the eating life you should have been living all along, and would have been living, if someone hadn't given you a different one, long before you were old enough or smart enough to know what they were doing to you.

And, in line with that, please keep one thing in mind: just because someone "**gives**" you something, that doesn't mean you have to "**keep**" it—unless you're talking about things like Christmas presents or birthday gifts.

I mean, when someone "gives" you a cold, what do you do: sit there and say, "Well, I guess I'd better 'take' whatever this cold is dishing out, because someone 'gave' it to me, and I don't want to hurt his feelings by not 'keeping' it"(?!)

Yeah, right: when someone "gives" you a cold, we know **exactly** what you'll be doing: taking an antihistamine for the sneezing and the runny nose; Visine for the watery eyes; Robitussin for the cough; aspirin for the fever; and so on.

In other words: **busting a gut to get rid of it**!

Why bring that up here?

For the reason I just mentioned: that just because someone **gave** you the eating life you're now living, that doesn't mean you have to **keep** it—especially if it's bringing you the same long-term misery a cold would, while giving you nothing in return except the minute's-worth of "joy" you get from that bag of cookies or that Caramel Frappuccino.

So what?

So, because someone **gave** you the eating life you're now living—because there's nothing "natural" about it, nothing you were **born** doing, like breathing— you won't be killing yourself by giving it **back** to them; trading it in for a **new** life, the life you should have been living all along, and would have been living if someone hadn't given you a different one, long before you were old enough or smart enough to know what they were doing to you.

And why is that line so important that we've brought it up twice in the last few minutes? Because it means it's **not your fault** that you eat the way you do, any more than it's a 30-year-old's fault if he smokes or drinks, since he was given those habits/addictions when he was still a child, and, therefore, incapable of knowing what the adults in his life were doing to him, until it was too late.

And, since we're on the subject, you really have to be amazed:

When an adult coaxes a child into letting the adult abuse the child **sexually**, we call that "statutory rape," and put that adult away for a long, long time, based on the fact that the child was too young to know what the adult was trying to do to him or her.

However, let that same adult coax a child into letting the adult abuse the child **chemically**—whether that chemical is nicotine, alcohol, sugar, or what-have-you—and we **don't** put that adult away for a long, long time. Oh no: instead, we give him **awards** for all that coaxing (something the advertising industry calls a "Clio") and pat ourselves on the back for allowing that abuser to exercise his First Amendment right to "free speech," while we bury—long before their time—the smokers, drinkers and obesics all that "free speech" has led to.

Like I say: you have to be amazed!

And now, back to our story.

So, again, it's not your fault that you eat the way you do, since you were given that way of eating long before you were old enough or smart enough to know what the big people were doing to you.

OK, fine.

However, that's no longer the case, is it?

Oh no: you're now **plenty** old enough and **plenty** smart enough to know what they did to you. Which means you're now plenty old enough and plenty smart enough to **un**do what they did to you.

Which is what we're here to help you do.

Does your typical abusive eater **want** to undo what the big people did to him; **want** to "cure" himself of cookies and candy and pancakes and pie?

Of course not.

Do smokers **want** to "cure" themselves of cigarettes; drinkers, of booze?

Of course not.

Those things have gotten their hooks so deeply into all of you that they've become a major part of your life.

No, check that: for many of you, they've **become** your life; everything else—work, home, school, etc.—has become merely "killing time" between Pop-tarts, Marlboros or "Breakfast Buds"!

Which means that **giving up** those things would be the same as giving up your **life**, which is an obvious no-no in anyone's book.

So, you don't give them up. Instead, you just keep on keeping on, giving in to every cookie, donut, and candy bar that calls your name.

And why shouldn't you? After all

• Unlike a generation or two ago, when the majority of Americans were either normal-sized or real close to it—which meant that oversized people ran a real risk of social rejection—that's no longer the case is it, because everywhere you look—at work, in stores, on TV, etc.—all you see are oversized people, so who's left to "cast the first stone?"

So, fear of social rejection has now gone the way of the dinosaur, as far as being a reason for doing something about body size.

• And if you're like most abusive eaters, you're not a bit concerned about what all that eating might be doing to your health, because, if you do run into trouble health-wise, the medical-pharmaceutical complex will be there to bail you out, the way they promise to in those TV ads.

Of course, that bailout won't come without a "price" (see Chapter 13), but, as with everything else in life, you'll "cross that bridge when you come to it." In other words, "nothing to see here"—especially if it might involve turning your back on that hot fudge brownie sundae every now and then.

• And you're not worried about losing your life-partner as a result of all that eating, because the thought of living alone is so horrific to most people that they'll put up with anything—endless eating, endless smoking, endless drinking, drug addiction, physical beatings, etc.—if that's what it takes to make sure there'll be someone to come home to at night.

• And you're not worried about losing your job because of all that eating, because a group of plus-sized people got together a while back and made their legislators pass laws that make it illegal to discriminate against someone based on body size. So **that** reason for doing something about that body size has gone by the wayside.

In short, no reason on Earth to change your eating—any more than smokers, drinkers, etc., have any reason to change what **they're** doing.

So, why do it?

Well, aside from the fact that all that eating is disabling and killing you—as surely as cigarettes and booze are disabling and killing **their** aficionados—because it shouldn't take more than **a week or two** to undo a **lifetime** of abusive eating.

Why such a short amount of time?

Because the thing that's making you eat—your Subconscious Mind—could care less what you ate 10 or 20 years ago. Oh no: as we've gone into in great detail, all it cares about is what you ate **yesterday**. Meaning that if you can string together a **couple of weeks'-worth of "yesterdays," free** of the endless eating of food in general and of certain foods in particular, it will stop making you hungry for those quantities and types of food. At which point, you'll be **cured** of those quantities and types of food, which is why we're here.

At the beginning of this book, we gave you one of our favorite sayings:

"If nothing changes, nothing changes."

Now, while that might sound like what my generation used to call "gobbledygook"—"Real profound, Dave: 'If nothing changes, nothing changes.' Come up with that all by yourself did you?!"—the fact is, it's **anything but**:

What it's saying is: your mind and body are set up to make whatever changes you "tell" them to make. Which means that, first, you have to "tell" your mind and body what you want them to change, which you do my making that change **consciously**. Once you do that, your mind and body will pick up on that change and make it **permanent**, without you having to give it a second thought.

So, that's what we'll be doing here: taking a week or two to have you **consciously** change the way you eat, so your mind and body can pick up on those changes and make them **permanent**, which will turn you into the normal eater you have no reason not to be.

Is that a long time: a week or two?

I don't know. What I do know, though, is that, if you're more than a few pounds oversized, we'd bet dollars-to-donuts you've given Sara and Ronald and the Doughboy at least one or two **decades**!

So what?

So, if you have one or two **decades** for **them**, please don't tell me you don't have one or two **weeks** for **us**—for you and me—to work together to **un**do what they've done to you!

And one very important point: as you take those one or two weeks to go from abusive eater to normal eater, never forget: if you don't like your life as a normal eater—don't like the fact that you have absolutely no desire for the foods you "couldn't live without" just a week or two before; don't like the fact that you're moving better, feeling better, looking better than you have in years; don't like the fact that you've most likely added weeks, months or even years to your life—if you don't like any of the things your new life has brought you, no problem: **go back to your old one**! It will still be there: Sara Lee will still be churning out cheesecakes; Ronald McDonald will still be hawking Deluxe Big Breakfasts; the Pillsbury Doughboy will still be spending millions of dollars every year, making 300-pounders accept, without question, that "Nothin' says lovin' like somethin' from the oven," though some might have a problem tying the word "lovin'" to products whose main claim to fame is that they make you fat, clog your arteries, rot your teeth, and get you addicted to them.

All we're saying is: would it really kill anyone to take a lousy week or two to see if maybe they could live their life **without** those things in it? I mean, if you can, you'll be "cured" of those things, and can start living the life that billions of normal eaters live every day; a life that's a **hundred** times better than the one you were living with all those things **in** it, no matter how much the food companies try to convince you it's not, and no matter how much short-term "joy" their cookies and donuts might have brought you.

And if, after those one or two weeks, you find you really **can't** live without those things in your life? No problem: **put them back in**! No one will stop you, because no one can.

Again: you can't give us "a week or two"?
Puh-lease!!

2

"Gotta Have It!"

So, we now know the way to get unnecessary quantities of **food in general** out of your life: by getting your Subconscious Mind to stop making you hungry for those quantities of food, in the name of satisfying its misguided "survival agenda"—which agenda, again, has absolutely nothing to do with a **physical** need for food, your **body's** need for food, no matter how much it might **feel** like it does—so you can start using up some of your **stored** calories for a change, instead of continually pouring tons of **new** calories down your throat.

However, before we go into the best ways of doing that, we have to tackle the other part of our equation: getting unnecessary quantities of **certain foods in particular** out of your life, with those certain foods in particular being, of course, foods you're chemically addicted to.

And why is that so important: to get chemically-addictive foods out of your life?

Because, by definition, once you start eating those foods, you can't stop. So the only way **to** stop is to **never start**!

Now, you'd think that admitting you're chemically addicted to something would be the easiest thing in the world for us humans to do; I mean, how much more evidence would you need than someone "scarfing down" a two-pound bag of Fun Size Snickers at a sitting; smokers lighting up a hundred times a day; drinkers downing a couple of "suitcases" of Bud Light after work.

Yes, you'd think that admitting you're chemically addicted to something would be the easiest thing in the world to do. And yet, it's not. Why not?

Because admitting that you're chemically addicted to something is to admit that the **smartest** things on the planet—that would be you and me—are being led around by the nose by the **dumbest** things on the planet—unless you think things like sugar molecules and nicotine molecules and alcohol molecules are, like,"mini-Einsteins"(!)—and no ego **I** know of is strong enough to admit that.

So, we don't. Instead, what we hear are:

"I can stop eating cookies/smoking/drinking anytime I want. I just choose not to—especially in 'social settings' where 'everyone' is eating cookies/smoking/drinking, so why shouldn't I?"

Answer: because you're not eating/smoking/drinking to "be sociable;" you're doing those things because you **have** to do them; because you're **addicted** to doing them, and the only way to **stop** doing them is to never **start**! Period!

Naturally, there will always be a few diehards who will **never** admit they're addicted to something; who will claim they **can** control their consumption, evidence be damned.

Well, for you folks, all we can say is: feel free to apply these other Tests for Addiction, and maybe **that** will convince you:

1) The first test, of course, is the one we just went into: if, once you start eating something, you can't stop until it's all gone—or until you pass out from the pain or the sugar rush—then you're addicted to that something.

The fact is: no one in the history of the world has ever been unable to stop eating an apple once he's started, whereas, if you had a dollar for every cookieholic who couldn't stop eating Oreos till they were all gone, you'd never have to work another day in your life!

2) If you can't even wait till you're through the supermarket checkout line to tear open your bag of something and start eating it, then you're addicted to that something.

No one in the history of the world has ever been unable to wait till he's back in the car to bite into an apple.

Side story:

When I was still single, I had a young lady over to my house, for coffee. That's right: coffee!

After I'd poured her a cup, she said, "Y'know, I think I'd like something sweet with this. Do you have, like, a cookie or something?"

"No," I replied, "I don't."

"Oh? You don't keep cookies in the house?"

At which point, I looked at her like she was from Mars:

"'Keep' cookies in the house?!" I thought to myself. *"'**Keep**' cookies?! Are you kidding?! I don't buy cookies to '**keep**' them; I buy cookies to **eat** them!*

*"I mean, those cookies are lucky if they **make** it to the house, forget 'keeping' them!"*

—but all I actually said was: "No, I don't keep cookies in the house."

Sound familiar?

3) If you get sexually aroused at the mere **thought** of a particular food, then you're addicted to that food. (Side note: you don't want to know what was going on between my legs, at one or two in the morning, as I got closer and closer to the store that sold my favorite chocolate chip coffee cake, especially if I'd "struck out" that night at the local "meet market!")

Again: no one in the history of the world has ever gotten sexually aroused by an apple.

Okay: one guy!

4) If you're driving home from work, and you're looking forward to some "goodie" you've carefully stashed away in the kitchen cupboard, only to find, when you get to that cupboard, that someone's gotten there before you and eaten the whole thing, and you find yourself spending the next hour trying to figure out the best way to **kill** that person, then you're addicted to that thing.

Again: no one in the history of the world has ever wanted to kill whoever ate the last apple!

I'm sure there are other tests for addiction, but those should get you started.

And please keep in mind: addiction never goes away. Once you're addicted to something, you're addicted to it forever; there's no "cure" for addiction, other than to get whatever it is you're addicted to out of your life, and never let it back in.

How do I know? Here's how:

In the early 1980's, I was working at a large, government installation in southern California, which had its own dining hall.

What the cooks would do is: they would prepare a certain amount of a dessert for the evening meal, with each person getting a single portion. Then, however much of the dessert was left over from that meal would be refrigerated, then hauled out the next day and put on a table in the center of the room, where you could now eat as much of it as you wanted.

Well, one day, the dessert happened to be something I really loved: coconut custard pie (not coconut **cream** pie; just coconut custard, sitting in a pie crust, in what looked to be a 2-foot-by-3-foot pan.)

Well, I finished my actual meal, took my plate to the center table, and loaded it "wall-to-wall" with that pie, then went back to my seat and ate every last drop of it.

At which point, I stood up, and was about to do the same thing all over again, when I stopped dead in my tracks: *"Hey, wait a minute:"* I thought to myself, *"If the two pounds of pie I just ate weren't enough to satisfy me—in fact, put not the slightest dent in my craving for it—what guarantee do I have that **another** two pounds will do the trick? Or two more after that? Or two more after that?"*

At which point, I put my plate back on the table, told my buddies to "wait right there," and went up to my room, where I pulled a half-eaten, 8-ounce Hershey bar out of my locker, brought it back to the dining room, and tossed it down in front of 425-pound Scotty—the largest member of our "fearsome foursome," which also included 350-pound Larry and 300-pound Butch, making me, at 5'10" and 275 pounds, the "thin man" of the group.

"What's this?" Scotty asked.

"I'm done with that."

"Done with what?"

"'Sweets.' Thanks to that coconut pie, it just became

painfully obvious to me that once I start eating stuff like that I can't stop. So, the only solution is to never start. So, enjoy every last drop of that Hershey bar."

"Thanks," Scotty said, "I will!"

And so it went, the afternoon of January 18, 1983.

So, how does that apply to addiction being uncurable?

Well, 22 years later, in August of 2005, my son and his fiancée were forced to evacuate New Orleans, just ahead of Hurricane Katrina, eventually winding up on our doorstep in California.

The fiancée, Marylyn—suffering, perhaps, from "cabin fever"—decided she wanted to bake something.

Which she did: this sort of "loaf," which was about an inch high and maybe four inches wide, and consisted of a thin crust, all around, with a filling of chopped walnuts and honey.

Now I knew I couldn't control my consumption of things like "cake"—something I'd finally admitted to myself 22 years earlier.

But this wasn't a "cake;" it was a "loaf."

"*Well, geez,*" I thought, "*anyone can handle a 'loaf!*'"

So, just to be sociable, I had a piece. And then another. And that was it—the first day.

The next day, I raced home from work, took the lid off the cake stand, cut myself a piece, buttered it, and ate it. Then did that all over again. And that was it —the second day.

The third day, I again raced home. But this time, the little loaf was nowhere to be seen—certainly not where it had been the day before.

I looked frantically through all the cupboards, but… no loaf!

At which point, my eyes happened to fall on our Simple Human garbage can.

"*Could it be?*" I wondered.

I sprung open the lid and sure enough, there it was: the rest of the little loaf!

Lucky for me, there wasn't more than a pound or two of coffee grounds on top of it, so it didn't take more than a minute or two to brush those grounds off, put the loaf on a plate, cut it up into a half-dozen pieces, butter those pieces and devour every last one of them!

You with me: **Twenty-two years** without anything even **close** to a cookie or a piece of cake. And yet, one taste of that "forbidden fruit" and it was "off to the races" again. It was if those 22 years had **never happened**; as if I was still in that dining hall, going back for plate after plate of coconut custard pie.

So, spare me the bullpuckey that it's possible to "get over" an addiction; to cure yourself of it, and to go back to eating whatever it was you were addicted to, but this time **not** "fall off the wagon."

Uh-uh; never gonna happen: once addicted, always addicted.

So, the only solution is to get that addictive something out of your life.

How?

Well, in a word: gradually.

Why gradually?

For the reasons we went into when we were talking about **mental** addiction: because your Subconscious Mind thinks you really do need those addictive somethings to survive. So, the minute you take those things away, your Subconscious Mind thinks you're trying to kill yourself, and it **can't let that happen**!

And the more **abruptly** you take them away—the more you go from hot fudge sundaes on Monday to watercress sandwiches on Tuesday—the more your Subconscious Mind will "get its back up," and the sooner you'll find those hot fudge sundaes right back in your life.

So, that's why we'll be doing this gradually—because we're here to cure you of an addiction, cure you of an eating disorder, not help you lose 10 pounds this week so you can gain back 20 the next! Again: **enough is enough** with that nonsense!

What we'll in fact be doing is the one thing you have to do, if this thing is going to work: fooling your Subconscious Mind into thinking nothing "fishy's" going on in your eating life, nothing that would make any alarm bells go off, which will **keep** it from "getting its back up;" will, if we do it right, **lull your Subconscious Mind to sleep**, so it has absolutely no reason to get you eating what it thinks you need to eat, to survive.

The way we'll be doing this is by having you go down what we call an "**addiction ladder**," with a highly-addictive food at the top of the ladder, and a totally non-addictive food at the bottom, and where every step in between contains a food that's just slightly less addictive than the one above it.

For example: let's say we want to get chocolate chip cookies out of your life. OK, so that would be the item at the top of the ladder.

What you would then do is: pick something that's **very similar** to chocolate chip cookies—say, the oatmeal-raisin variety—and eat those without limit, if necessary, day after day.

And what will this do?

Just one thing: it will put **time** between you and your last chocolate chip cookie.

Why is that so important?

Because that's all you **have** to do, to get chocolate chip cookies out of your life.

Why?

Because every day you do without chocolate chip cookies and make it to the next day "tells" your Subconscious Mind that you **didn't** need those cookies to make it to the next day, so it no longer has any reason to make you hungry for them. So it doesn't.

And, if you're not hungry for chocolate chip cookies—not "craving" them—why would you eat them?

Answer: you wouldn't.

So you don't.

At which point, you'll be "cured" of chocolate chip cookies—which, again, have absolutely no business being in your life, any more than cigarettes and booze have any business being in **their** addicts' lives, and would never have been in your life in the first place if someone hadn't put them there, long before you were old enough or smart enough to know what they were doing to you.

Again, do abusive eaters "want" to cure themselves of chocolate chip cookies?

Of course not: their whole life revolves around the fact that "you're only here once," so, as the old Schlitz commercial told us, you have to "grab for all the gusto you can." And, if that gusto just happens to involve chocolate chip cookies, or pancakes-and-maple syrup, or pie à la mode, or so on and so on, then that's what you'll be grabbing for—the same way smokers grab for cigarettes, and drinkers, booze.

OK, fine.

But, if we may be so bold: as much "gusto" as all those cookies and pancakes might be giving you, they can't hold a candle to the **true** "gusto" of **not being enslaved by them**!

How do we know?

Because **we** stopped being enslaved by them almost 40 years ago, and haven't regretted, for a minute, that those things are no longer in our life; are no longer **ruling** our life.

So, before you say, "If I can't have those things in my life, I'd **rather not live**!" take the couple of weeks it will take to get those things **out** of your life and then get back to me.

Look: at one point in my life, I swore I "couldn't live" without a couple of bacon-egg-and-cheese biscuits in the morning. Or, later in the day, a Carl's, Jr. Western Bacon Cheeseburger, which, in addition to the bacon and the cheeseburger, featured a couple of delicious onion rings and a fantastic barbecue sauce. Or anything Baskin-Robbins, Haagen-Dasz, or Ben & Jerry put out. Or…well, you get the idea.

And yet, those things that I "couldn't live without" are now nowhere to be seen in my life—and haven't been for decades—and there are no words to express how little I miss them, and how glad and how thankful I am to be **rid** of them!

Which is why we're here: to help **you** get rid of them, and to replace them with some of the most marvelous, non-addictive foods in the universe.

And now, back to the ladder…

So, we get chocolate chip cookies out of our lives by replacing them with the oatmeal-raisin variety, and eating the latter for as long as it takes to get the craving for the former to vanish.

Why oatmeal-raisin cookies?

For this reason:

The fact is: your Subconscious Mind's "eyesight" is not all that good.

In the current example, it's trying to get you eating chocolate chip cookies, which are brown cookies with dark chunks in them.

And what are oatmeal-raisin cookies?

Of course: brown cookies with dark chunks in them.

So, when your Subconscious Mind "looks out" to see if you're eating what it's trying to get you to eat, and it sees that you are, in fact, eating "brown cookies with dark chunks in them," its "eyesight" is not good enough to tell which "brown cookies with dark chunks in them" those are. So, it has "no choice" but to give you the **benefit of the doubt**, and assume that you're eating the chocolate chip cookies it **wants** you to eat, rather then the oatmeal-raisin variety you're **actually** eating; which means it won't be getting its back up and won't be making you break down walls to get the chocolate chip kind.

At which point, chocolate chip cookies will be out of your life, and you **won't miss them**!

The next step?

Of course: getting the oatmeal-raisin cookies out of your life.

And how do we do that?

Of course, by proceeding to the next step down the ladder, where you find something slightly less addictive than oatmeal-raisin cookies—say, Nabisco's Vanilla Wafers (OK: 'Nilla Wafers! Sheesh!)—which you then eat—without limit, if necessary—until all desire for oatmeal-raisin cookies has vanished.

At which point, you proceed to the next step down the ladder, where you find, say, Wheat Thins, which you eat—without limit, if necessary, and with maybe a little butter or cheese on them—until you've lost all desire for 'Nilla Wafers.

At which point, you proceed to the bottom of the ladder, where you find any number of great-tasting, low-calorie crackers: Triscuits, Wasa Crispbread, Mary's Gone Crackers, etc., which you then eat, without limit, until all desire for Wheat Thins has vanished.

"But I don't **want** to eat Triscuits or Crispbreads without limit!"

BINGO! Cured of chocolate chip cookies—and of everything in between—without your Subconscious Mind having realized, anywhere along the way, that that's what you were doing, which meant it had no reason to **stop** you! So, it didn't.

"OK. But won't eating all those cookies and wafers and Wheat Thins put some weight on me?"

They might. But that's not the point here.

The point here is: we're trying to get addictive substances out of your life. And the way you do that is by putting time between you and your last cookie, your last Pop-tart, etc., because, again, every day you do without those cookies and Pop-tarts and make it to the next day "tells" your Subconscious Mind that you **didn't** need that garbage to make it from one day to the next, so it stops making you hungry for it.

And, if you're not hungry for it….well, again, this is where we came in.

So, don't worry about any extra weight those cookies, wafers, etc., might put on you, as you proceed down the ladder. Once you hit bottom, and no longer have any desire for those things, whatever weight they might have put on will quickly disappear, since there will be nothing left to sustain it.

At which point, you can tackle the next thing you're addicted to—say, ice cream.

OK, so we have ice cream at the top of the ladder.

The step below it?

Well, why not: fruit-at-the-bottom yogurt, which you eat—without limit, if necessary—until all desire for ice cream has vanished.

At which point, you proceed to the next step down the ladder, where you find **plain** yogurt, with **you** now adding the fruit—bananas, strawberries, raspberries, etc.—so there's no added sugar, like there is with the fruit-at-the-bottom kind.

The next step down?

Of course: just plain yogurt, which you eat without limit, if necessary.

"But I don't **want** to eat plain yogurt without limit!"

BINGO: Cured of ice cream—and of everything in between—without your Subconscious Mind having the slightest idea that's what you were doing.

And so it goes, getting one addictive food after another out of your life—the same way they're out of the life of **every** non-addict—by setting up an "addiction ladder" for every one of them, and reminding yourself, as often as necessary, that those things would never have been in your life in the first place if someone hadn't put them there, long before you were old enough or smart enough to know what they were doing to you, and, quite frankly, if a million forces in your life didn't **keep** them there:
- Your Mommy—in person or in your head
- Your Subconscious Mind
- Food company advertising
- The chemicals in those foods
- Your friends and family
- and *ad infinitum*.

So, that's Step One: getting chemically-addictive foods out of your life, and doing so in such a way that the thing that makes you do everything you do—your Subconscious Mind—has no idea that's what you've been doing. Which means it has no reason to stop you.

Which means we can now proceed to Step Two: getting unnecessary quantities of **food in general** out of your life.

3

The Cherry on Top

So, you've gotten—or are in the process of getting—addictive foods out of your life.

Which means we can now proceed to the next step in the program: getting unnecessary quantities of **food in general** out of your life, the same way they're out of the life of every normal eater on this planet.

And how do we do that; how do we get unnecessary quantities of food in general out of your life if, like most abusive eaters, your main goal is to see how much food you can get **into** your life every day, the same way smokers try to see how many cigarettes they can get into their lives, and ditto for drinkers and booze?

So, how do we do that; how do we get food **out** of your life—or at least off center-stage in your life—when all you want to do is keep as much of it as possible **in** your life?

Of course: the same way we do everything: by being aware of the way your Subconscious Mind works and then using that knowledge to get it to leave you alone.

Again, every sandwich, every cookie you have on Monday "tells" your Subconscious Mind to make you hungry for that sandwich, that cookie on Tuesday, thinking that sandwich, that cookie was the **reason** you got to Tuesday.

And please keep in mind: your Subconscious Mind has no idea—and could care less, even if it did—what all the sandwiches and cookies it's been making you eat have been doing to you **physically**. Oh no: its only job is to get you **eating** those sandwiches, those cookies, thinking that's what you **have** to do, to make it from one day to the next.

It doesn't know—and doesn't care—that you may already have a thousand sandwiches or a thousand cookies "in storage." Oh no: if you have a sandwich, a cookie on Monday and make it to Tuesday, it thinks that sandwich, that cookie was the **reason** you made it to Tuesday. And, since its only job is to get you to Wednesday…well, you know the drill.

However, even though **it** doesn't know and doesn't care what all those sandwiches and cookies have been doing to you physically, that doesn't mean that **you** shouldn't—especially since you're the one "wearing" them!

So, don't be afraid to tell yourself, every time you get hungry for a sandwich or a cookie: "Hey, wait a minute: I already have a thousand sandwiches/a thousand cookies 'in storage.' So, how badly could I possibly need this **new** one?"

Answer: you couldn't.

Which means you can take a pass on that sandwich, that cookie, without killing yourself.

And what happens if you take a pass on that sandwich, that cookie?

Of course: that "tells" your Subconscious Mind that you didn't need that sandwich, that cookie, to make it from one day to the next, so it will stop making you hungry for them.

And, if you're not hungry for them…

So, that's what we'll be doing here: getting unnecessary sandwiches, cookies, etc., out of your life, the same way they're out of the lives of every normal eater on the planet.

And how will we be doing that?

Again: by getting rid of the thing that's keeping them **in** your life: the hunger, the craving you have for those things, which, again, if you're more than a few pounds oversized, has absolutely nothing to do with a **physical** need for those things, your **body's** need for those things, no matter how much it might feel like it does.

And how will we be getting rid of those phony hunger pangs; how will we be getting your Subconscious Mind to stop creating them?

Of course, by not giving it the "fuel" it needs, to create those hunger pangs. In other words, by "withdrawing" from unnecessary quantities of food in general, the same way you did—or are in the process of doing—with certain foods in particular.

The fact is, every time you get a hunger pang, you have a choice:

• you can ignore it, let it pass; or
• you can satisfy it with what your Subconscious Mind wants you to satisfy it with; or
• you can satisfy it with "something else."

Obviously, the best thing you could do would be to ignore the hunger pang altogether; to simply let it pass.

And why is that the best thing you can do?

Because that will tell your Subconscious Mind in **no uncertain terms** that you **didn't** need whatever it was making you hungry for—making you crave—to make it from one day to the next, which will make it **stop** making you hungry for that thing in the shortest possible time.

And do keep in mind: if you don't give in to your Subconscious Mind for a time or two, eventually it will stop trying, since, unlike the majority of the humans it lives in, it knows how dumb it is to "keep beating a dead horse"—a phenomenon wonderfully illustrated by an episode of a very popular TV show from the 1990's: "Mad About You," starring Paul Reiser, as Paul Buchman, and Helen Hunt, as his wife, Jamie.

The episode, titled "The Conversation" (Season 6, Episode 9, available on YouTube), deals with Paul and Jamie trying to figure out the best way to get their baby to sleep on its own; that is, to get the baby to stop crying for mommy or daddy every time it's left alone—obviously, after making sure all other possible reasons for the baby crying—hunger, diaper rash, the room being too hot or too cold, etc.—have been checked off the list.

The point of the episode is: your first instinct, when you hear your baby crying, is to go pick it up and comfort it. However, if you do that, then the baby will never **stop** crying when it's left alone, leaving open the possibility that it might **never** learn to sleep alone (or, in later life, "stand" alone.)

So, what do you do?

Well, in Paul and Jamie's case, you have a conversation—standing, then sitting, outside the baby's room—agonizing over, "Do we go in there or not? Do we go for the temporary 'fix'—getting the baby to stop crying—in exchange for no long-term solution to the problem? Or do we 'tough it out:' enduring the misery of 'abandoning' our baby in its 'time of need,' to give ourselves the chance, at least, of solving the problem once and for all?"

The conclusion? You "bite the bullet:" you let the baby cry itself out—going in, if at all, to comfort the baby **verbally**, but not **physically** (by picking it up.) Once the baby realizes it's not going to "die" without mommy and daddy picking it up all the time—while still realizing that mommy and daddy are there for it in a "pinch"—it quickly turns its attention to other things, and the problem is solved—if not the first night, then the second or the third.

By the way, even though you now know how the whole thing turns out, we'd still recommend watching the actual episode, since it was not only one of the best episodes in TV history, but had the unusual feature of having been done in a single "take;" that is, unlike normal, filmed TV shows, where the camera stops every now and then for various reasons, this episode was filmed all at one time—something which is riffed on quite cleverly in the show's closing credits.

And why is this TV episode relevant here?

Because, like Paul and Jamie's baby, your Subconscious Mind received most of its programming in your first year of life. Meaning that it is basically an infant. Meaning that it reacts to things the way an infant would: throwing a temper tantrum if it doesn't get what it wants—in this case, if you don't feed it what it's asking for.

So that, like Paul and Jamie's baby, if you **keep** feeding it what it's asking for (if you keep "picking it up"), it will never **stop** asking for it. Whereas, if you can "gut it out"—if you can let the phony hunger pang pass unsatisfied, which it will, in 10 or 15 minutes—your Subconscious Mind will **stop** creating such things for you, since no rational creature keeps doing something if that something isn't producing the results the creature is going for!

And if your Subconscious Mind is not creating phony hunger pangs for you, why would you eat anything?

Answer: you wouldn't.

So that's why "letting the hunger pang pass unsatisfied" is your best bet, because doing so will eventually "erase" all phony hunger pangs from your life, the same way your first-grade teacher erased everything on her blackboard at the end of each day.

However, if that's not possible—if the pain is simply too great to be ignored—then the next best thing is to give yourself as much non-addictive food as it takes to make the hunger pang go away, then giving the next phony hunger pang a little less, and so on and so on, until the phony hunger pangs stop coming altogether.

At which point you will be cured of unnecessary quantities of **food in general**—which, when combined with being cured of **addictive** foods, will mean that you can simply start living your life as a normal eater.

And, if we have to say it a thousand times, we'll say it a thousand times, because it's that important: if you're not happy with your life as a normal eater; not happy that you're looking better, moving better, feeling better than you have in years; not happy that you've most likely kicked a host of obesity-related diseases out the door: diabetes, heart disease, high blood pressure, any number of cancers, etc.—if you're not happy with all the things having pancakes and Pop-tarts out of your life bring you, no problem: **put them back in again**! They're not going anywhere!

All we're saying is: just take the week or two it will take to get those things out of your life; to see what your life might be like without those things in it.

And, if you don't like your life without those things in it?

No problem: **put them back in again**! No one will stop you, because no one can!

So, do it. Take the simple steps outlined in this book to get unnecessary quantities of food in general—and of certain foods in particular—out of your life.

And one of the best ways of doing that is: every time a hunger pang comes along, just tell yourself:

"OK, I've got this hunger pang. It feels real—feels like my body really needs some food—but I know it can't be real, because my body already has a ton of food in storage.

"So I know it's not my body creating this hunger pang for me; it's my Subconscious Mind, in its never-ending quest to get me eating the same things today that I ate yesterday, thinking that's what I need to do, to survive. Except…I don't.

"So I'm either going to ignore this hunger pang and let it pass—knowing that I'm not going to be killing myself if I do—or I'm going to make it go away with however much good food that might take.

"Either way, that will put me one day closer to never being bothered by phony hunger pangs again, until the inevitable day that they vanish from my life altogether, and I can just eat **good food** when I'm **really hungry**, which, like my fellow normal eaters, will be 'almost never.'"

And while you're on the road to that normal-eating life, here are some fun things to think about…

4

"Hard-hat Area"

It would be nice if we could just toss a couple thousand tons of bricks and mortar, lumber and nails, shingles and drywall, pipes and paint up in the air and have it come down a house!

It would be nice, but it's never going to happen.

Why not?

Because houses aren't built that way.

No: houses are built a brick at a time, a 2-by-4 at a time, with every brick and every 2-by-4 moving you one step closer to a finished house; a house you can live in for the rest of your life.

And so it is with normal eating: it would be nice if you could just go to sleep an abusive eater and wake up a normal one; go from wanting to eat **everything** in sight to wanting to eat **nothing** in sight; go from a stomach that cries out to be fed **all** the time to a stomach that cries out to be fed **none** of the time.

It would be nice, but it's never going to happen.

Why not?

Because a normal-eating life isn't built that way.

No: it's built the same way you build a house: one "brick," one "2-by-4" at a time—until, one day, it's finished.

And what are those "bricks," those "2-by-4's," where a normal-eating life is concerned?

Of course: each "brick," each "2-by-4" is a food you get out of your life—telling yourself, with every one of those foods: "If I don't like my life without this food in it, I can always put it back in again. It's not going anywhere. I'm just going to take a week or two to see what my life might be like **without** this food in it, since, if I can get along without this food in it—a food that would never have been in my life in the first place if someone hadn't put it there, long before I was old enough or smart enough to know what they were doing to me—then I'll be just that much better off; that much closer to eating the way normal people eat.

"And again: if I don't like my life without this food in it, I'll simply put it back in."

So, that's what we'll be doing here: getting one food after another out of your life, replacing it with as much good food as you like, until you've gotten unnecessary quantities of food in general—and of certain foods in particular—out of your life completely. At which point, your "house"—your normal-eating life—will have been built, and you can simply walk through the front door every day and live in it.

The question, of course, is: **why** can't you change your eating overnight? I mean, that's what all the diet-pushers expect you to do—go from hot fudge sundaes on Monday to carrot sticks on Tuesday—so why is that so difficult?

And the answer is simple: Because, as we've said, the thing inside your head that makes you eat has too much time and energy invested in those hot fudge sundaes, syrup-soaked pancakes, etc., to let you get rid of them willy-nilly; thinks you need those things to survive, so that, when you suddenly take them away, it thinks you're trying to kill yourself, and it can't let that happen.

Which is why we take them away gradually—one food at a time—until they're all gone, but without our Subconscious Mind ever suspecting that's what we were doing, so it never has any reason to stop us.

The question, of course, is: why is that so important—to turn yourself into a normal-eater?

And the answer is simple: because

No normal eater in the history of the world has ever been one ounce oversized and none ever will be!

That's kind of important, so let me repeat it:

No normal eater in the history of the world has ever been one ounce oversized and none ever will be!

True, abusive eaters on their way to **becoming** normal eaters—and maybe for a little while after they get there—might still be oversized. But that oversize won't last—can't last—because there will be nothing left to sustain it.

So, that's why it's so important to become a normal eater: because it's the only thing you **have** to do, to put your oversize behind you.

So, that's what we'll be doing here: helping you build that normal-eating life—one "brick," one "2-by-4" at a time.

Of course, there are those who ask, "Why do I have to take the time and trouble to become a 'normal eater'? Why can't I just go on a diet, knock off a few pounds, and be done with it?"

To which we say: good question. And here's a good answer: No matter what diet I ever went on—and I went on a lot!—under no circumstances would I ever go to my closet and toss out all the extra-large clothing there.

Why not?

Because I knew I could **never guarantee** that whatever weight the diet **took** off would **stay** off!

And when I finally took the other route; when I turned myself into a normal eater?

Then, no hesitation whatsoever in getting rid of those oversized clothes, since I knew I would never "backslide;" would never be that size again.

That's why it's so important to become a normal eater, because that's the only way you can **cure** yourself of that excess bodysize, once and for all!

And to help keep you going on your path to normal eating, just remind yourself, as often as necessary: Rome wasn't built in a day, but eventually it **did get built**!

5

Normal Eater

Since the whole purpose of this book is to turn you into a normal eater—to take you from the DreamWorld-today/NightmareWorld-tomorrow that is the hallmark of abusive eating—because of that, this might be a good time to flesh out what a "normal eater" actually is.

Well, among other things:

1) A normal eater is one of the 7 billion people on this planet whose life is **not** based around food; who **doesn't** spend every waking moment thinking about it, talking about it, reading about it, buying it, preparing it, eating it, etc.—the same way a non-smoker is one of the 7 billion people on this planet whose life is **not** based around setting fire to a dead plant a hundred times a day, and a non-drinker is one of the 7 billion people on this planet whose life is **not** based around going to bed drunk every night.

Why bring that up—the "7 billion people" thing?

Simply to show you that, if you do turn yourself into a normal eater, it's not exactly like you'll be all alone out there, which, yes, can be a little scary.

2) A normal eater is someone who sees food for what it is, what it was intended to be: a source of simple, yet pleasant, nutrition—and not what it was never intended to be: a source of

- Love: "Nothin' says lovin' like somethin' from the oven."
- Reward: "Finish all your homework and you can have some milk and cookies."
- Sport: "Whoever eats the most food at Golden Corral, Ryan's Steakhouse, Hometown Buffet, etc., 'wins'"(?!)
- Comfort: "Were those boys mean to you? Here, have a piece of cake."
- Punishment: "If you don't finish every last drop of those pancakes, you're not going to the beach/the movies/the ballgame/etc., with us!"
- And *ad infinitum*

3) A normal eater is someone whose Subconscious Mind is **not** calling out for food at all hours of the day and night, especially when there's no physical need for any.

4) A normal eater is someone who can go down a supermarket's ice cream aisle, cookie aisle, candy aisle, etc., and feel not the slightest longing for any of those things.

5) When it comes to a "treat" or "dessert," a normal eater thinks: an apple, an orange, a slice of melon, a peach, a plum, a nectarine, cherries, etc., not apple pie, orange sherbet, peach cobbler, cherries jubilee, and the like.

6) A normal eater doesn't use the tiniest of hunger pangs as a reason for launching into a 10-course meal, when a couple of crackers or a handful of nuts would have easily done the trick.

7) An abusive eater finishes a meal and says, "How soon till we can eat again?"

A normal eater finishes a meal and says, "How soon till I can I walk this all off?"

So that's what a normal eater is, and what we're here to help you turn yourself into—to your unending gain, and, quite frankly, the food companies' unending loss.

Oh…poor little food companies!

6
By Design

Before we get too far along in this program, we'd like to remind you of something we brought up in *Walk Yourself Thin* and *Walk Yourself Fit*, and ask you to burn it into your brain:

> The more you eat, the more you
> **want** to eat,
> **need** to eat,
> **can** eat.
>
> The less you eat, the less you
> **want** to eat,
> **need** to eat,
> **can** eat.

These are Laws of Nature; they can't be broken. You get along on less by "training" your body to get along on less, not by stuffing yourself. The more you eat today, the more you'll want tomorrow; the less you eat today, the less you'll want tomorrow.

Or, in broader terms:

> **You design your own tomorrows
> by the things you do today.**

It seems to be human nature—except for the most responsible among us—to think we'll never have to "pay a price" for the things we do; that we can eat whatever we want, smoke whatever we want, drink whatever we want, etc., and never suffer any consequences because of it—a state of mind the food companies, tobacco companies and booze companies of the world couldn't be more thrilled to hear about!

And, of course, everyone who falls for such nonsense will continue to be victimized by it.

So, why not take a minute and realize that everything you do **does** have consequences—that you **are** going to have to "pay a price" someday—and start living like you will?

In other words, start living a bit more of an **examined** life—where you **stop** before plunging in mindlessly to that hot fudge sundae, that bag of cookies, that chocolate cake, etc., and, instead, ask yourself the magic question:

"Yes, I can eat that sundae, those cookies, that cake. And yes, it will bring me a moment's-worth of 'joy.' But it's not like I'm not going to wind up '**paying**' for that 'joy,' in terms of added bodysize, increased risk to my health, the need to put out money for larger clothes, etc.

"So, the question is: is that moment of 'joy' worth the days and months of 'misery' it will lead to, when the fact is, I'm only eating that sundae, those cookies, that cake out of habit, or to satisfy an addiction, and not because I have any **physical** need for any of those things? Which means I won't be starving myself to death if I don't have those things, since my body already has hundreds, if not thousands, of those things in storage, which it would be more than happy to bring **out** of storage and **use**, if I'd just let it. In other words, if I'd just stop adding to it.

"So why don't I try **that** for a change, instead of constantly giving in to every cookie and donut that calls out my name?"

Will this work, the first time you try it?

Probably not.

I mean, I don't know about you, but I can't remember a **thing** that worked the way I wanted it to, the first time I tried it.

And yet, because I kept trying, eventually the whole exercise did pay off.

So, why not at least **try** this little trick, to see what life-changing payoff **you** eventually get?

7

Scary Movie No. 53

As we've said previously: we're here to let you know why you eat the way you do, so you can change that way of eating, if you want.

Of course, there are people out there who'd rather you **not** have all this knowledge; who are perfectly happy with you **never** knowing why you eat the way you do.

Those people are called "food companies" (though it's a stretch to classify what many of them sell as "food!")

Like any company, their job is to make money: if they make enough of it, they survive; if they don't, they don't.

Obviously, they make their money by selling you food—and, just as obviously, the more of it the better. So, anything that threatens those food sales—like this book—is something they have to stop, and **stop now**!

And what's the best way of doing that?

Of course: the way governments, politicians, corporations, parents, etc., get us doing anything: by **scaring the bejeezus out of us!**

Which is why, within weeks of this program seeing the light of day, you can expect to see—in tabloids and, perhaps, some of the more mainstream media as well—something along the lines of

"Woman Starves to Death on Rives Program!"

And why will you see these stories?

Because, as we've said previously, food companies need you eating **all** the time, rather than virtually **none** of the time, the way normal eaters eat, and those companies simply can't let that enormous gap go unfilled.

And how do they get you eating all the time?

Of course: by frightening you into believing that, if you're **not** eating all the time, you'll starve to death—conveniently forgetting that, if you're more than a few pounds oversized, you already have weeks'-, months'-, or even years'-worth of food in storage, so how badly could you possibly need any **new** food?!

Answer: you couldn't.

But will the article tell you that?

Not on your life!

Why not?

Because it's the food companies who'll be paying to have that article written and run—the same way virtually every corporation pays the media, in one way or another, to have its message written and run—and the last thing they want to hear out of you is questions like: "Hey, wait a minute: I already have a year's-worth of food in storage. So, how am I going to starve to death by taking a 'pass' on those brownies/pancakes/Pop-tarts/etc.?"

No, if there's one thing you'll never see in any article about the "dangers" of this program, it will be the part about "How can I possibly starve to death when I already have a ton of stored food to draw on?"

Answer: you couldn't.

Of course, this whole argument is irrelevant, since, in just a minute, we'll be giving you a thousand foods you **can** eat all day. Which means that, if someone does starve to death on this program, it certainly wasn't because of anything **we** told them!

Again, the only reason we bring this up is to alert you to what most likely will be coming: an article or articles intended to frighten you away from what we're telling you here and get you back to the pancakes and Pop-tarts those fearmongers **have** to sell you, if they want to keep themselves in Cadillacs and Cessnas.

Again: knowledge is power, and knowing that such articles will be coming will give you the power to ignore them when they do.

So, that's our mission: to let you know, as far as eating is concerned,

- How you got here
- Why you stay here
- How to get out of here, if, at some point in time, you decide you've "had enough;" that your abusive eating is just not "doing it" for you anymore, and you're looking for a change.

And what change can we offer you? Simply this: we can take you from a life of nonstop eating to a life where eating will be the **last** thing on your mind; where your body **stops** calling out for food every minute you're awake, the way it doesn't call out for food every minute **normal** eaters are awake.

That's it. That's the life we can take you to. And all you have to do is start.

And now, as promised, the "thousand foods" you can eat without limit:

Apples and oranges and tangerines and grapefruits and pineapples and peaches and pears and nectarines and plums and cherries and grapes and blueberries and blackberries and strawberries and raspberries and bananas and mangoes and papayas and cantaloupes and watermelons and honeydew melons and almonds and pistachios and walnuts and lettuce and tomatoes and cucumbers and carrots and celery and bell peppers and onions and cabbage and olives and eggplants and mushrooms and spinach and cauliflower and broccoli and Brussels sprouts and peas and green beans and squash and rice and parsnips and rutabaga and avocados and artichokes and hummus and tahini and tikka masala and pickles and eggs and cheese and crackers and rice and quinoa and cottage cheese and…well, you get the idea.

Again, if someone manages to starve to death, given that they can eat every one of those things till the cows come home, then the problems they're dealing with involve a lot more than **eating**!

8

The Greatest Gift

Each day, every one of us is given the greatest gift we'll ever get:

That Day!

Don't think it's the greatest gift? Thought the "greatest gift" would be measured in things like "horsepower," or "beam length," or "square feet," or "carats," or "karats"?

Well, go ask Abe Lincoln or Franklin Roosevelt or Howard Hughes or J. P. Morgan how many sports cars, yachts, mansions, diamond necklaces, gold bracelets, etc. they'd give up, just to have one more day on Earth, and then get back to me!

No: the bumper sticker we saw the other day says it all:

"The best things in life aren't things."

In other words, nothing we **get** in life can hold a candle to **life, itself!**

So the only question left is: what do we do with this "greatest gift"?

Well, if you're addicted to nicotine, you fill that greatest gift with as many cigarettes as you can, thereby tossing that greatest gift straight in the trash by destroying the only body you'll ever have.

If you're addicted to alcohol, you fill that greatest gift with as much booze as you can—again: destroying the only body you'll ever get.

If you're addicted to sugar—or to eating endless quantities of food—then that's what you'll fill your greatest gift with—and, like smokers and drinkers, disable and kill yourself long before there was any need to.

So there it is: every day, you're faced with a choice: fill that greatest gift with all manner of garbage, thereby handing your life over to Sara Lee, Anheuser-Busch, or Philip Morris.

Or

Stop filling it with garbage, and start living the life you were **put** here to live, rather than the one Sara and Anheuser and Philip **need** you to live.

That's it; that's your choice.

Obviously, we hope you'll follow our lead and choose to get unnecessary quantities of food in general—and of certain foods in particular—out of your life, so that you can **make the most** of the gift you were given, rather than continuing to treat it as a piece of junk.

9

Annie

And now, the best tip you'll ever get:

Obviously, this program is based on getting your Subconscious Mind out of your life—at least, as a destructive force in your life; getting it to stop making you hungry for things you have no physical need for.

Thus, anything that can **keep** your Subconscious Mind at bay—**keep** it from creating phony hunger pangs for you, to satisfy its whacked-out "survival agenda"—is to be welcomed and cherished.

We've already told you that you have to do this thing **gradually**; have to make a **gradual** transition from abusive eater to normal eater, because that's the only way you can make your Subconscious Mind think nothing "fishy" is going on; nothing that will sabotage its built-in program to get you eating the same things today that you ate yesterday—thinking that's what you need to eat to stay alive, even though you don't—because, if it does think that, then it will get its back up, and sabotage **your** program to get those things **out** of your life.

Thus, the one thing you must never do—even though you might want to—is announce to your Subconscious Mind, either out loud or internally:

"That's it! I'm done with cookies and candy and everything like them! From now on, it's just cucumbers and celery sticks!"

And why must you never do that?

Because the minute your Subconscious Mind "hears" that, it's going to say, "Oh yeah? Well, we'll see about that!" and, within a half-hour, tops, you'll find yourself sitting in front of the biggest bag of Chips Ahoy or Snickers bars you've ever seen!

Why?

Because, again, your Subconscious Mind thinks those cookies and candy bars are what's keeping you alive. So, the minute you tell it that you're getting those things out of your life, it thinks you're trying to kill yourself, and it can't let that happen.

And yet, those are the very things you do have to get out of your life, if you're ever going to become—or return to being—the normal eater you have no reason **not** to be.

So, how do we reconcile those two things; how do we get those things out of your life without your Subconscious Mind getting in the way?

Here's how:

Instead of announcing—out loud or in your head: "That's it! I'm done with cookies and candy forever!"—what you tell your Subconscious Mind instead is: "You and I are going to be sitting down and having the biggest bag of chocolate chip cookies the world has ever seen! We're going to be eating those cookies from morning till night! We're going to be having the biggest cookie party in history! That's right! And we're going to be doing all that…**tomorrow**!

"Today, however, what we'll be having is a crisp salad, with tomatoes and cucumbers and celery and a mix of lettuces and a delightful vinaigrette dressing, and with maybe an assortment of cheeses and crackers on the side.

"But tomorrow? **Look out, world**: we're going to be having so many cookies Nabisco won't have to worry about paying the rent till the year 2050!

"Today, however, just let me at that salad!"

And what will that do?

Simply this: it will get your Subconscious Mind saying to itself: "Gee, I'd really like to get her eating those chocolate chip cookies **today**. However, 'tomorrow' is **not all that far away**. So, as long as I know she'll be eating those cookies tomorrow, I'll **leave her alone today**."

Which it does.

And when "tomorrow" comes?

Of course: you do the same thing all over again:

"Man, I can't wait to polish off those 50 dozen chocolate chip cookies I've got sitting in the cupboard, and will definitely do so...**tomorrow**!

"Today, however, what I'll be 'polishing off' is a 6-inch sub, with maybe a small bag of chips, and an apple for dessert.

"But tomorrow? Look out cookies, 'cause **here I come!**"

And again, your Subconscious Mind will respond with: "Well, as long as she's going to be eating those cookies tomorrow, I'll leave her alone today."

And when tomorrow comes...well, you know the drill.

And what will all this "tomorrowing" do?

Of course: the only thing you have to do, to get unnecessary quantities and types of food out of your life: put **time** between you and your last cookie, your last pancake, your last Pop-tart, your last piece of cake, and so on, because every day you do without those things and make it to the next day "tells" your Subconscious Mind that you **didn't** need those things to make it to the next day, so it will stop making you hungry for them—until, in a couple of **weeks'**-worth of "tomorrows," that hunger will vanish altogether. And, if you're not hungry for something—not craving it—why would you eat it?

Answer: you wouldn't.

At which point, you'll be **cured** of all those things, and all because you "told" your Subconscious Mind that it wasn't going to have to **give up** any of those things; that you were going to be having them all without limit…**tomorrow**!

And once again, you're going to have to take our word for it: as much "joy" as **eating** all those cookies and pancakes and Pop-tarts might be bringing you, it can't hold a candle to the true joy of being **free** of them. Which is exactly what you'll discover when you arrive at that "promised land."

So, do it.

And by the way, the reason this "tomorrowing" is the best tip you'll ever get is because it can be applied anywhere:

Every time you want to do something but know you shouldn't—like putting out money you really can't spare for something you really don't need, or not getting your house organized when you know you should, or binge-watching TV when there are a million more important things you know you should be doing—just tell yourself: "I'm definitely going to be doing that something—putting out that money; leaving my house a mess; binge-watching TV…**tomorrow**! Today, however, what I'll be doing is **keeping that money in my pocket**, **getting** my house in order, **doing** one of those million important things.

"But tomorrow? Look out! I'll be spending money like a drunken sailor, leaving my house an unholy mess, watching TV till my eyes fall out!

"Today, however, what I'll be doing is: keeping that money in the bank; making my house an example to the world; doing everything **but** bingeing on TV."

And, of course, when "tomorrow" comes, you do the same thing all over again.

And what will that do?

Of course: every day you **don't** spend money unnecessarily, **do** get your house organized, **don't** binge-watch TV, etc., brings those things closer and closer to becoming **habits**—the same way not eating cookies or pancakes or Pop-tarts day after day becomes a habit, so you simply stop eating them, and do so without giving the whole thing a second thought. And anytime you can make something a habit—especially a good thing—so that doing it becomes automatic, that can't help but put you one step closer to your best possible life.

So have fun with this. Pick out your own personal things to apply the "tomorrow" principle to. And then let us know how it turns out.

10

Bobby and Dale

Obviously, we're all born "wet behind the ears"—that is, naïve to the ways of the world—meaning that it's not all that far-fetched to look at life, itself, as little more than a series of getting "dry" behind the ears; in other words, having our eyes opened to realities that, until that moment in time, we never knew existed.

Naturally, I can't recall my first "drying" experience, but I can, in fact, recall at least one very vividly:

In my family, if someone mentioned "food treat," everyone knew what they were talking about: candy, cookies, donuts, brownies, pie a la mode, etc.

Well, one day, when I was walking home from school with a friend of mine, Bobby Finkel, we came upon a bakery. Since I happened to have a little extra cash in my pocket, I said, "Hey, Bobby, let's go in here; my treat."

So, in we went, to be met by the most dazzling array of goodies you've ever seen: chocolate éclairs, Napoleons, lemon meringue tarts, 7-layer cakes; double-fudge cupcakes; cherry Danish; apple Danish; cheese Danish; and *ad infinitum*.

"So, what will you gentlemen be having today?" the nice lady asked.

"Go ahead," I said to Bobby, "anything you want," anticipating he'd ask for an éclair, or a custard donut.

Well, Bobby looked through all the cases, then happened to notice some wire bins behind the clerk.

At which point, he made his decision: "I think I'll have an onion roll."

At which point, my Earth came to a screeching halt!

"Uh, Bobby, I don't think you understand: I said you could have anything you wanted."

"I know," he replied, "and I want an onion roll."

Allow me to explain: at that time, an "onion roll," in our neighborhood, meant an 8-inch wide, 1-inch thick, totally-unsweet bread product, with moist onion flakes and poppyseeds pressed into its upper surface (think "full moon" here, only brown). Total calorie count: 100, tops—or about what was in **each bite** of the chocolate éclair **I** ordered!

And it was at that very moment, in my eighth year on this planet, that I first came to realize that there were people here who were different than me; who, when confronted with an "ocean" of what I just assumed **everyone** considered "treats," would instead opt for something that **no one** I knew would have attached that word to—a fact which, as it happens, came in very handy a few years later, when I finally decided to get those things out of my own life: knowing that there was at least one person on this planet who could turn his nose up at all those sweets—and be none the worse for wear because of it—meant that I could, too. And did.

Naturally, I don't think I have to tell you what "onion-roll Bobby" looked like: thin as a rail—though that didn't keep him from being one of the strongest, toughest kids in school.

And "éclair Dave"? Well, if I'd had the word "Goodyear" printed on my side, no one would have blinked!

And yet, thanks to Bobby, I eventually did give up all those treats, and managed to get just about as thin as he was.

Until a couple of decades later, when those "treats" had somehow worked their way back into my life:

Was working at a TV station in Los Angeles, in the early 1970's, in an office I shared with a guy named Dale Dodd.

Well, one afternoon, Dale and I were up in the second-floor break room, where I tore open a two-pack of fudge cookies and offered him one. To which he replied: "No, thanks: I don't eat sweets."

At which point, my Earth once again stopped turning, as it had 20 years before, leaving me standing there in stunned disbelief: "*'Don't eat sweets'*"? I thought. "*'Don't eat sweets'? Crikey: 'sweets' are **all** I eat—or at least all I **want** to eat!*"

I mean, if it weren't for me, the "roach coach" that came to the station every day—with its cookies and brownies and donuts and tea cakes and candy bars and you-name-it—would have long since gone out of business!

"*Don't eat sweets*"?! I thought to myself. "*Are you crazy? Don't you know what you're missing?!*"

And the answer to that is: No: Dale didn't know what he was "missing"—any more than Bobby did, some 20 years earlier—because, to "miss" something, you have to have had it in your life in the first place, which neither of these guys ever did.

Why bring that up here?

Because there's a chance that you've never run across your own "Bobby Finkel," or your own "Dale Dodd;" that you don't know there are people out there who could "care less" about the things you (and I) "can't live without."

So what?

So, like me, once you do know those people exist, it should make it that much easier to become one of them; to get sweets out of your life for good, the same way they were "out" of Bobby's and Dale's lives.

And, as it happens: once you do get them out of your life, your desire for them will drop to zero, like it was for Bobby and Dale.

And, if you have no desire for something, why would you eat it?

Answer: you wouldn't. And won't.

At which point, you will be "cured" of that something, and will begin looking at an **apple** as as big a treat as apple **pie** used to be; at a **banana** as as big a treat as a banana **split** used to be; and, yes: at an **onion** roll as as big a treat as a **jelly** roll used to be.

In other words, you will "become" Bobby Finkel; you will "become" Dale Dodd, which is all you have to do to get garbage foods out of your life and keep them out. Which is all you have to do to get down to normal size. Which, in case you missed it, is what we're all about!

11

Scrubbing Bubbles

As an aside…

The problem with brainwashing is, if it's done right—and, given we humans' desperate need to see everything in black-and-white: "This is definitely good;" "This is definitely bad," rather than in endless shades of stomach-churning gray—given all that, it's almost impossible **not** to do it right—if brainwashing is done right, the brainwashee has no idea what's been done to him. He accepts whatever the brainwasher tells him as "fact," and, as a result, will defend that "fact" to the death, if necessary.

Which is how we get treated to things like "Breakfast is the most important meal of the day," which most people take as a nutritional "fact." Which is fine, except when you dig a little deeper, and discover that this "fact" started out in life as nothing more than an advertising line, to help a couple of guys in the 19th century sell their recently-invented breakfast cereal, and then again during World War II, to do the same thing.

Doesn't matter: the line has become so engrained in everyone's psyche that they accept its validity without question—using it, in the case of your typical abusive eater, to justify a breakfast of eggs and bacon and sausage and muffins and hash browns and pancakes and cinnamon rolls and you-name-it, on the basis that, if breakfast is, in fact, "the most important meal of the day," then the **bigger** the breakfast, the more "important" it **must be**!

Which is how you wind up with 300-pounders in McDonald's, day after day, having no qualms whatsoever about eating all those things; shoving thousands of calories down their throat, then spending the rest of the day burning off absolutely none of those calories, so what reason was there to have them in the first place—aside from the "fact" that "Breakfast is the most important meal of the day"?!

Or things like: "It's a crime to waste food," and its first-cousin: "'Cleaning your plate' is, at all times, a virtue."

Which is how you wind up with people like the 250-pound lady we saw at an all-you-can-eat restaurant, using her fork to scrape every last molecule of food from the plate she had just finished (her first? her fifth? her 20th??) onto the 10 pounds of food on the plate she was about to dig into; someone who had not the slightest need for **any** of those molecules, and yet was unable to discard so much as a **single one of them** because of the "fact" that "it's a crime to waste food" and "cleaning your plate is always a virtue."

Or, on a different note: a presidential candidate, stumping for votes from a certain audience, knowing how the honest, hard-working members of that audience felt about a certain group of people, then appealing to that feeling by creating what he referred to as a "Welfare Queen:" an imaginary Black lady, cheating the government out of money by driving her Cadillac to one welfare office after another, collecting one check after another, totaling, what, a thousand dollars a month?, with that same candidate, after becoming president, then pouring **billions** of dollars into the hands of his defense-contractor buddies, for an anti-ballistic-missile system known as the "Strategic Defense Initiative" (or, as everyone called it, "Star Wars"), a system so complicated—and so politically-charged—that it never had the slightest chance of getting off the ground (and never did), meaning that we might just as well have flushed all those billions of dollars down the toilet, for all the good they were going to do us.

But did this president call **that** "welfare"? Of course not.

Why not?

Because the defense industry has lots of money to get people elected, which the made-up "Welfare Queen" never did.

The result? That president turning the mythical "Welfare Queen" into a "**fact**," and getting the brainwashed public to hiss and boo, every time her name came up, for "taking a hard-earned thousand dollars out of their pockets," while, at the same time, giving the defense industry a "pass" for cheating those same people out of **billions** of dollars, dollars that could have gone into building or repairing the schools their children went to, the roads they drove on, the bridges they crossed, etc.

That's right: one (made-up) Black woman—**one**—cheating those millions of people out of at most a thousand dollars a month—or, what, a couple of pennies apiece?—and yet she's the villain, while the defense industry, cheating them out of billions, are the good guys!

As we've said elsewhere: You have to be amazed!

So, how do you cure things like that?

I don't know, since the brainwashee accepts everything the brainwasher tells him as **fact**—because he **wants** to, **needs** to—and how do you argue with "facts"?

All we can say is: ask yourself, every time you run across one of these "facts," if there might not be an ulterior motive going on here:

• breakfast food companies trying to sell you more product;

• mothers whose families lived through the Great Depression or the Second World War, where food could be hard to come by, making sure that the food in front of you today is as precious to you—and thus not to be "wasted"—as it was to your grandparents and great-grandparents, 80 or 90 years ago, even though whatever food we're talking about here was already "wasted" long before **you** got hold of it, since the hamburger you're eating can never again become a cow, the bread you're eating can never go back to being stalks of wheat, blowing in the wind, etc. Meaning that, whether you eat the hamburger, the bread, or throw them in the trash (i.e., "waste" them), the result is the same, so why eat them—and add more material to your fat stores—because of the ridiculous—though totally unquestioned—"fact" that "it's a crime to waste food"?

• politicians trying to distract you from what they're really doing, by telling you to "Look over there!"

• and *ad infinitum*.

Other than that, when it comes to overcoming brainwashing, it looks like all we can do is cross our fingers and hope for the best!

12

Perry Como

We hear it all the time: "I have a hundred pounds to lose. It's hopeless!"

And you're right: if you did have a hundred pounds to lose, it **would** be hopeless.

But you **don't** have a hundred pounds to lose. No one does. In fact, no one ever did.

"But—"

What you "have" to lose is: **one ounce**! Once you've lost that one ounce, then we can talk about a second ounce, then a third, etc., until, one day, you've lost a **hundred pounds-worth of ounces**, but without that figure—"100 pounds"—ever rearing its ugly head.

The problem here is: you're looking at that 100 pounds as if it's something that has to be lost **all at once**; and you're right: if that were the case, the situation would be hopeless.

But that 100 pounds **doesn't** have to be lost all at once—in fact, **can't** be lost all at once. So, every time you think that's the way you **have** to lose it—because that's the way you **want** to lose it—you'll never lose a thing.

Which is why we tell you: the only thing you **have** to lose is "one ounce." Once you've lost that one ounce, then we can talk about a second ounce, then a third, etc.

Yes, we know, this is just a variation of the old saw: "A journey of a thousand miles begins with a single step." But just because that "saw" is **old** doesn't mean it isn't **true**. The fact is, a journey of a thousand miles **does** begin with a single step—always has and always will—and so does your journey down to normal body size.

So, forget that "100 pounds," and just concentrate on losing that **one ounce**—because until you lose that single ounce, everything beyond it is irrelevant, whereas once you do lose that single ounce, the rest is a piece of cake!

13

"It's Coming!"

If there's one thing you can bet the house on, it's that a drug will be coming along any day now that will simply blow the weight off you, without you having to so much as lift a finger or give up a single cookie.

How do we know?

Because there's just too much money to be made from such a drug for it to stay **un**invented for very much longer.

Of course, this new drug won't come without a ton of side effects, like the ones you see advertised on TV, where the drug companies spend the first 10 seconds of their commercial telling you all the wonderful things their drug will be doing for you, and the last 20 seconds telling you how their drug will basically **kill** you!

Which won't matter a bit, because the minute you hear those first 10 seconds, you'll be out the door, making a beeline to your doctor or pharmacy, to get yourself a bottle of the new drug!

How do we know?

Because we've been through this before, back in the 1990's, when a drug called Fen-Phen hit the market and took off like a rocket!

And it didn't matter when someone at the Food and Drug Administration finally decided to take an in-depth look at Fen-Phen and discovered that that particular combination of drugs—**Fen**fluramine and **Phen**termine—just happened to be
- turning people's heart valves into oatmeal, and
- blowing up their lungs,

which was leading to a nasty little side effect we call: "**death**!"

Which news, of course, found all those oversized people running right to their trash cans and dumping whatever tablets they had left, then dashing off a glowing letter to the FDA, thanking them for saving their lives!

Yeah, right: If Hell hath no fury like a woman scorned, then they'd have to invent a new **category** of fury for the way those oversizeds and obesics reacted to having their favorite drug taken away from them: threatening to **kill** the people who were trying to keep **them** from getting killed!

And when these protestors were told, again, that the drug could kill them, their response was always the same: "We don't care! It works! That's all we care about! Why don't you let **me** decide whether I want to live or die? I mean, it's **my freakin' life**!"

And why were these people so in love with a drug that they'd risk death to take it?

Because, like they said, it worked—giving us what came to be known as the "Fen-Phen Effect;" to wit:

I had a business associate, Tom, who was as abusive an eater as they come: couldn't wait to get out of bed in the morning to start eating; drove to work eating, stopping only long enough to pick up a dozen donuts for "the crew" (yeah, right!); snacked all morning; then had a five-course lunch, complete with dessert; then…well, you get the picture.

And then one day…nothing! No donuts, no dessert—nothing!

So I asked him what happened.

His response: "Fen-Phen happened."

"'Fen-Phen'?"

"Yep: take a pill in the morning, and then…well, let me put it this way, Dave: you plop down a plate of anything in front of me, put a gun to my head, and tell me, 'If you don't eat that food, I'm going to blow your brains out,' my only response would be, 'Well then, you'd better start "blowing," because I'm not touching a drop of that garbage!'"

That's right: the number-one eater in the world—the guy who'd rather not go on living if he couldn't have his afternoon bag of Cheetos—that same guy now choosing to die, rather than put one forkful of food in his mouth!

That was Fen-Phen!

And that was why its fans threatened to **kill** the guys who'd taken it off the market, even though the drug they wanted back was killing **them**!

And why did these people do that? Why were they threatening to kill the guys who were **saving** their lives?

Because Fen-Phen was the drug they'd all dreamed of: something that would completely kill their appetite without making them have to bite a bullet to do so, and that would blow the weight off them without asking them to move so much as an **eyebrow** muscle—all of which was just too appealing to these lifelong "foodaholics" for them to let the drug go off the market without a fight.

So, they didn't, even though, eventually, it did.

Why bring that up here?

For this reason:

No matter what weight-loss drugs the pharmaceutical companies come up with, every one of them is going to have side effects—many of them deadly, as drug after drug has shown: Fen-Phen; Vioxx; Avandia; Actos; Celebrex; Yaz/Yasmin/Ocella; and *ad infinitum*.

Yes, it's comforting to think that some runny-nosed PhD on the fourth floor of the Pfizer Building knows more about our bodies than Whoever **gave** us these bodies; that that "lab rat" can somehow "sidestep" the body's incredible complexity—where everything interacts with everything else—and simply zero in on just one aspect of that body without having an effect on any of the others.

Yes, it's comforting—it's what every overweight and obesic is **praying** will happen—but, as drug after drug has shown us, it's never **going** to happen, so you might just as well stop praying.

Which means you'll have a choice when that drug finally hits the market and starts showing up on TV: listen to the first 10 seconds of the commercial, then fly out the door to get you some,

Or…

Stay put on the couch—after those first 10 seconds have run their course—and listen to the last part of the commercial, where they'll be telling you—in the **sweetest, most upbeat voice you've ever heard**—how their drug will kill you!

It's your choice.

And, if you do stay on the couch, please remember to congratulate yourself, a year or two later, when the drug gets pulled off the market for injuring and killing more people than you can count.

Of course, the wonderful thing here is, you don't have to **take** Fen-Phen—or anything like it—to get the Fen-Phen **Effect**! That's right: you can get that effect simply by doing this program.

How so?

This so:

The "Fen" part of Fen-Phen (fenfluramine) works by making your brain pump out a chemical that signals "fullness," which, of course, "kills" your hunger, your appetite, so the **last** thing you want to do is eat (P. S. The other part of Fen-Phen—phentermine—works by increasing your metabolic rate, so you burn a few more calories per hour. But that's not nearly as important as the appetite-suppression that the "Fen" part gives you, because who cares how many calories the "Phen" part might be helping you **burn** if you never want to **eat** any?!)

So, all we have to do, to get the Fen-Phen Effect, is make sure our brains are doing what Fen-Phen makes them do: pump out enough of that hunger-killing chemical that we feel full all the time.

And can we do that?

Yes, we can—and without taking a single pill:

As we said earlier: when you eat something on Monday and make it to Tuesday, your Subconscious Mind thinks that something was the **reason** you made it to Tuesday. And, since its only job is to get you to Wednesday, that would seem to make its job rather simple: just get you eating that same thing all over again.

Which it does, by creating a hunger, a craving for that thing that's all-but-impossible to resist. And one of the ways it **creates** that hunger is by cutting off the flow of that hunger-killing chemical in your brain.

"It's Coming!" 79

Obviously, if your hunger is not being "killed," that must mean it's very much "alive," which means you're very much going to satisfy it, since that's what we humans are hardwired to do.

And if you eat even **more** on Tuesday than you did on Monday, then your Subconscious Mind will have to make you even **hungrier** on Wednesday than it did on Tuesday, which means it will have to hold back even **more** hunger-killing chemical on Wednesday than it did on Tuesday.

And so on and so on, until, eventually, it winds up holding back **all** the hunger-killing chemical and you're never **not** hungry. Which means you're never **not eating**.

Which is how you get a nation of 300- and 400-pounders eating plate after plate of food, with none of them ever feeling "full."

Why?

Because their Subconscious Mind makes sure that the chemical that would **tell** them they're full might just as well be on Jupiter!

The solution?

Obviously: get your Subconscious Mind to stop doing that; to stop holding back the flow of that hunger-killing chemical; get that chemical once again flooding your brain after even the tiniest of meals.

In other words: do what Fen-Phen does.

How?

Well, again: the more you eat on Monday, the more your Subconscious Mind cuts off the flow of that hunger-killing chemical on Tuesday. Which gives us the solution: start eating less and less each day.

Again, if you're more than a few pounds oversized, you obviously have no **physical** need for all those calories, no matter how much it **feels** like you do. So you won't be killing yourself by withholding a few, every now and then.

And what will that do?

Well, when you **stop** eating something on Monday—replacing it with either nothing, or with a reasonable amount of actual food (apples, oranges, nuts, etc.)—your Subconscious Mind will have no reason to make you **hungry** for that something on Tuesday. Which means it will have no reason to block the flow of that hunger-killing chemical. Which means that chemical will start flowing again; and the more it flows, the less hungry you'll be, so the less you'll eat. Until you'll eventually feel full on the amount of food that normal eaters feel full on every day, which is: next-to-nothing.

Will this happen instantaneously, the way it does with Fen-Phen?

No: it could take a week or two, since most of you will be making the transition from nonstop garbage to normal amounts of good food **gradually**.

But the fact is: it **will happen**—and without you having to worry about dropping dead from heart failure or a blown-out lung!

So, there's your choice: take the new drug that's coming out (or go back to Fen-Phen; it's available on the Internet), and worry every day about the drug killing you.

Or

Eat a little bit less every day and eventually experience the exact same appetite suppression that Fen-Phen would give you—for the exact same reason—but without any of the nasty side effects.

That's it; that's your choice.

Hope you'll choose wisely.

14

Dead-end Street

By now, I assume everyone has seen the Snickers commercials (if you haven't, they're all on YouTube), that tell us: "You're not you when you're hungry," and that show how otherwise-levelheaded people turn into insufferable "divas" (portrayed by the likes of Aretha Franklin, Betty White, Liza Minnelli, et. al.) when they're hungry, and how all it would take, to get the Real You back, would be a bite of a Snickers bar.

Which it does—for about a half-hour.

And then what?

And then the "nightmare:"

You always have a certain amount of sugar floating around in your blood: about a quarter-teaspoon per cup of blood. Your body's cells use that sugar for energy, which helps keep you on an even keel.

What you've also got is a little guy inside your head, sitting on the banks of the Red River (a.k.a., your bloodstream) keeping tabs on how much sugar is in that river.

As long as it stays at that quarter-teaspoon-per-cup level, the little guy stays put.

However, the minute the little guy sees your blood-sugar level falling **below** that quarter-teaspoon per cup, he springs into action, doing whatever he can to get you eating something—increasing your stomach contractions, making you impossible to live with, etc.—since he knows that that's all it will take to get your blood-sugar level back up to normal again.

So, you eat something—if you're a normal eater, maybe a cracker or two, or a piece of toast, or an apple or an orange—all of which gets carried from your stomach to your liver, where it gets turned into glucose, which is the only sugar your cells can use, with that glucose then getting poured from the liver back into your bloodstream—thereby getting your blood-sugar level back up to normal or a little above—and then on to your cells.

Now, as it happens, that glucose can't get into your body's cells on its own; it needs something to "push" it in—a chemical we call "insulin," made by something called the "pancreas," a little organ that sits right behind your stomach.

If you've eaten a "reasonable" amount of food, your liver will turn that into a "reasonable" amount of glucose, meaning that your pancreas only has to put out a "reasonable" amount of insulin to push that glucose into your cells.

Once that newly-minted insulin has pushed enough sugar into your cells to get your blood-sugar level back down to normal, your liver then destroys it.

Why?

Because if that extra insulin **stayed** in your bloodstream, it would **keep** pushing sugar into your cells—I mean, **it** has no idea what a normal blood-sugar level is; its only job is to push sugar into cells—until you wound up back where you started: sitting there with low blood sugar, meaning the little guy in your head has to make you hungry and irritable all over again, to get you eating again.

However, what if, instead of a "reasonable" amount of food to ward off low blood sugar—say a single bite of a Snickers bar—you wind up downing the **whole bar**? Then what?

Then, instead of the "trickle" of glucose coming out of your liver, which it would if you'd satisfied your hunger pangs with a **small** bite of that Snickers bar, what you get instead is a "**tsunami**" of glucose pouring out of your liver, which means your pancreas has to put out a **boatload** of insulin to take care of that sugar.

Again, if your liver is able to destroy all the extra insulin that might still be hanging around after all that excess sugar has been pushed into cells and your blood-sugar level has returned to normal, then "no sweat": no low blood sugar, no return of the hunger pangs, and no "diva" problem.

But what if it can't? What if there's so much extra insulin floating around that your liver **can't** destroy it all in time?

Well, then that insulin **keeps** pushing sugar out of your bloodstream and into your cells, so that your blood-sugar level goes **below** that normal quarter-teaspoon-per-cup, leading, once again, to a situation of **low** blood sugar (what the fancy folks call "hypoglycemia"), which once again forces the little guy in your head to get off his duff and start creating **more** hunger pangs for you. Which you satisfy with **more** Snickers bars, which will overload your bloodstream with **more** glucose and **more** insulin, leading to a vicious cycle that (potentially) has no end: eat a Snickers bar, get temporary relief from your low blood sugar, but suffer an even worse bout of low blood sugar—and, with it, increased hunger pangs and cravings—

when your body gets overwhelmed by that first Snickers bar, leading to a need for a second Snickers bar, then a third, then a fourth and *ad infinitum*—obviously, much to the joy of the Snickers **company**!

So there you have it: the Snickers bar that was supposed to kill your hunger and make you **less** of a "diva"—which it did, for about a half-hour—in fact leaving you **hungrier** and **more** of a "diva" in the **next** half-hour—and the half-hour after that, and the half-hour after that…—a little factoid the Snickers company conveniently forgets to tell you about.

And not only that, but, when you do get to that second or third Snickers bar, and the extra insulin it leads to can no longer push all that sugar into your body's "**regular**" cells, because those cells are "**full**," it takes it to the only place that can and will accept it, and virtually without limit: your fat pads—leading, before very long, to you-know-what!

So, what to do?

Well, now that you know what happens every time you dump a load of sugar into your body—the launching of a vicious cycle of hunger-killing, followed by bigger hunger creation; the need for bigger hunger-killing, which leads to even bigger hunger creation; and so on—you can avoid all that by switching over to foods that **don't** do that—things like apples and oranges and salads and crackers and nuts and *ad infinitum*.

Naturally, the Snickers company—and Sara Lee and Tony the Tiger and Betty Crocker and Mrs. Butterworth and Dunkin Donuts and the Keebler Elves and the Pillsbury Doughboy and Baskin-Robbins—won't be all that **happy** that you've switched.

However, just one question: Is that really why you were put on this planet—to make **them** happy?!

15

"Play Ball!"

When I was nine, my family moved house—from a neighborhood where **no one** played sports to one where **everyone** did! Which I knew meant that I'd better get good at sports myself—and **really fast**—or I'd soon be spending a lot of time with my thumb up my a**!

As it happens, it didn't take long for me to figure out that the easiest way to get good at something was to simply watch people who were already good at it and then try to copy them.

Luckily, the city I grew up in—Detroit, Michigan—had no shortage of sports figures who were "already good" at their craft, including future Hall-of-Famers like Al Kaline in baseball, Gordie Howe in hockey, and Bobby Layne in football.

So, that's what I did: watched the way Al Kaline went after a fly ball; caught it; threw it (with his arm fully extended); hit it; etc.—and then tried to do all those things as closely to the way he did them as I could.

And the same thing with Gordie Howe—the way he skated; carried his stick; handled the puck; took a shot; etc.

And ditto with Bobby Layne and throwing a football.

Which, after a few months, is how I managed to get **really good** at all those things!

No, not Al Kaline-good, or Gordie Howe-good, or Bobby Layne-good, else you'd be visiting **me** in some Hall of Fame somewhere.

No, I never got that good. But I did get good enough that, when it came time to choose up sides for a neighborhood baseball or football game, I was almost always the first one picked (P. S. There was virtually no such thing as "organized sports" [Little League baseball, Pop Warner football, etc.] in the area of Detroit I grew up in, so we had to be content with neighborhood or playground pick-up games.)

Anyway, that's the way I learned to do things: by watching others do them and then trying to do them the same way—a way of learning so obvious that I just assumed that's the way everyone did it.

Until years later, when I had my **own** nine-year-old, and I was coaching him and his buddies in Little League, where we would often get matched against a team that had an outstanding player—a shortstop; second baseman; outfielder; etc.—and I'd try to get my own kids to watch that outstanding player, so they could learn from him, the same way I had learned from outstanding players when I was their age.

And did they?

Ha!: my kids would look at me like I was from Mars, and would just keep throwing their gloves at each other, or playing with their trading cards, or giving each other "noogies," or doing whatever it was they were doing at that moment to make sure they didn't do what I had asked them to do, what I knew they'd benefit from doing.

As an aside: I'm not sure what had happened, in the 35 years since **I** was nine, to make this group of children so different than the ones I grew up with, but something did, with the main difference being the fact that my generation would play baseball any time and any place—the street, the playground, etc.—whereas, if these kids were not participating in an "organized" game—with uniforms, umpires, official fields, snack bars, etc.—they wouldn't even get **near** a baseball, forget about playing a **game**!—but, whatever it was that led to such a change, I'm not all that sure it was such a good thing.

Obviously, however, it's way too late to change any of that, so I guess we just soldier on.

The reason I mention all the above, of course, is that, even if no one nowadays sees the value in learning from watching others, that doesn't make it any less valid a way of living, of making one's life better.

Why bring that up here?

Because every day, you have a choice:

You can keep watching oversized people eating sandwiches they have no need for, cookies they have no need for, donuts they have no need for, etc., and copy **them**;

Or

You can watch the way normal eaters eat—a salad here, a piece of fruit there, etc.—and copy **them** for a change—copy the people who are **doing it right**—the same way I copied Al and Gordie and Bobby in the long ago, which helped me go from total clod to neighborhood "star!"

That's it; that's your choice: keep thinking those oversizers are doing nothing wrong with their 1,000-calorie breakfasts, 2,000-calorie lunches, and 3,000-calorie dinners, when—News Flash!—they already have a million calories in storage;

Or

Look at the normal eaters around you and model your life after **them** instead, to your unending gain and the Big Food billionaires' unending loss.

Your move.

16

Crime of the Century

While there are obviously a million things, over the last 100 years, that could qualify as the Crime of the Century—Hitler's Holocaust; Josef Stalin murdering millions of his own people; the Rwanda genocide; etc.—when it comes to the Crime of the Century as far as losing bodysize is concerned, there can be only one candidate:

The Invention of the TV Remote.

Why?

Oh, not for the reason you might be thinking: the fact that we're no longer burning the calories we used to burn, walking back and forth to the TV, to change the channel, adjust the volume, fix the Horizontal or the Vertical, etc.

No, as important as the loss of that calorie-burning might be, it pales in comparison to the real reason the invention of the TV remote qualifies as the Crime of the Century, which is:

Because it changes things in the blink of an eye.

Crime of the Century 89

So what?

So this: Because **one** thing can be changed in the blink of an eye, we suddenly don't understand why **everything** can't be changed that way—including our bodies!

When that doesn't happen—since it can't—we simply throw up our hands, come down with a cookie in one and a caramel macchiato in the other, and go our merry way.

How to get around that?

Easy: realize that your body doesn't work the way your TV does, and interact with your body the way **it** works, not the way you **wish** it would work.

Specifically, every time you look at yourself in the mirror, remind yourself:

"Oh yeah: those fat pads weren't put there to vanish at the click of a button. They were put there to keep me going in times of famine, which happened to my great-great-…-great grandfather a thousand years ago, and yesterday afternoon in Ethiopia.

"And even though **I** would like those fat pads to go in the blink of an eye, those **fat pads** have no idea what I'd 'like.' All they 'know' is what they're hard-wired to do: conserve fat at all costs, so they can keep me going as long as they can, when there's suddenly no food around!

"So, the **last** thing I can expect them to do—in fact, would **want** them to do—is vanish at the drop of a hat, since, if there really were a famine happening, the next thing vanishing at the drop of a hat would be **me**!"

In other words: realize that, where survival is concerned, your body sees those fat pads as an asset, not a liability, and, like any asset, it will do everything in its power to conserve them—which means: fighting your every attempt to get rid of them.

So, please keep that in mind when you've cut your eating down to next-to-nothing (in other words, when you're eating the way normal eaters eat), or when you're walking a zillion miles a day, and yet nothing seems to be happening to those fat pads.

The fact is: it's not "supposed" to happen, so stop getting angry and disappointed when it doesn't, and just be thankful for any little thing that does!

And, speaking of that: as we told you—in *Walk Yourself Thin* and *Walk Yourself Fit*—under the heading: "Murphy's Law of Body Size Reduction":

Wherever you really want the bodysize to leave, that's where it won't!

Why bring that up here?

For this reason: when you look at yourself in the mirror, your eyes will always go to the part of your body where you really want the size to leave— meaning, for most of you, your "love handles" and belly fat.

So what?

So, when it looks like those two areas aren't losing **anything**, day after day, you'll just throw up your hands, with an "Oh what's the use?", and go back to eating everything in sight.

You'll never look at the areas that **are** losing bodysize— your ribs, your face, your thighs, your calves, etc.—because, quite frankly, you don't care what's happening there.

And because of that, you wind up giving up on a program that was working quite well, thank you, just not as quickly as you wanted it to, and not in the places you were wanting it to work.

The solution?

Easy: instead of spending all your time looking at areas where the program seems to **not** be working (even though it is, just not fast enough to suit you), instead concentrate on those areas that **are** getting smaller every day—your ribcage, your back, your calves, etc.—and forget about those areas that apparently aren't.

To repeat, bodysize leaves so slowly, no matter what bodysize-reduction program you're on, that, as we brought up in this book's predecessors, you're better off if you **never** expect to see it leave. That way you'll never get disappointed.

So, that's Step One here.

But there's another downside to bodysize not leaving in the blink of an eye:

We'd bet dollars-to-donuts that, at some point in your life, you dieted or exercised like crazy on a Monday, then weighed yourself or looked at yourself in the mirror on Tuesday, only to discover: no change.

So, you "doubled" your dieting or exercise on Tuesday, then ran to the mirror again on Wednesday, to once again discover: no change.

So, you "tripled" your dieting or exercise on Wednesday, with the exact same results: no change on Thursday.

At which point, you said, "Oh, to Hell with it," and went out and had a hot fudge sundae.

The next day, you again looked at yourself in the mirror, anticipating the worst—either no change or an **increase** in body size, thanks to that sundae—only to find: you'd **lost** some size!

"Ohmigod," you said, "can this really be happening? Have I finally discovered the secret of the universe: that the key to bodysize loss is **not** dieting and exercise, but **hot fudge sundaes**?!

"I mean, what else can I think: I dieted and exercised like crazy on Monday, and Tuesday, and Wednesday, and got nothing for it in return. But one hot fudge sundae on Thursday, and bingo: **bodysize gone on Friday**!

"So, isn't it obvious: when it comes to losing bodysize, dieting and exercise are a waste of time, but **hot fudge sundaes** are where it's at?!"

Which is why you had another hot fudge sundae on Friday and, sure enough, took off even **more** bodysize by Saturday!

"Wow," you said, "I was right!"

Which is why you had no problem repeating the process all over again on Saturday, then racing to the mirror on Sunday—to see how much **more** bodysize you'd lost—only to discover: you hadn't lost any; in fact, may have **gained** an ounce or two.

"Oh well, just a temporary glitch. Another hot fudge sundae today and I'll be right as rain by tomorrow."

Except, when "tomorrow" comes, you're not. In fact, you've once again gone "the other way."

What went wrong? Why did your Hot Fudge Sundae Diet suddenly "go south" on you?

Easy: as we said: just because **one** thing in your life can be changed instantaneously, that doesn't mean that **everything** can—especially your body size.

Obviously, if your body were a TV, it could be changed instantaneously. But your body is **not** a TV; it's a living organism, and living organisms operate a whole lot differently than 60-inch flatscreens:

The fact is: no matter how much dieting or exercise you do, it can take your body a **hundred steps** to **process** any changes—each of which steps takes time, and a lot of it.

Which is why whatever dieting or exercise you do on Monday—and that you'd like to have show up on your body 10 minutes after you finish—won't, in fact, be showing up **anywhere** till **Thursday** or **Friday**! Which means you'll be facing terminal disappointment every time you think it **will**.

So, don't expect it.

Instead, every time you go out for a walk—or cut your eating way back—on a Monday, tell yourself: "Oh yeah: whatever I do today won't be showing up on me till Thursday or Friday, so I'm not expecting it to. Because if I do expect it to, I'll just get disappointed and quit, and **then** where will I be?"

Answer: nowhere, as far as losing bodysize is concerned.

So keep that concept firmly in mind, every time you take steps to change your body size: whatever you do will take at least three or four days to "bear fruit," which should get rid of any false expectations of how quickly those changes should show up. Which should keep you from quitting, thereby leaving those extra inches of bodysize on **you**, instead of on the street, track, or treadmill, where they "belong."

17

Night and Day

As we've said elsewhere, you have to be amazed:

Tell someone you can cure them of cancer—a deadly disease—but it might take a long time, and there might be some painful moments along the way, and the response you'll get is: "Doc, you take as long as you need. And, as far as the pain is concerned, well, we'll just cross that bridge when we come to it."

On the other hand, tell someone you can cure them of obesity—an equally-deadly disease—and the response you'll get is: "OK—as long as it doesn't take more than a half-hour, and as long as I don't have to give up any of the foods I love"(!)

Why is that? Why such a difference?

Easy: because food companies

- Have access to sugar, so they can keep people addicted to their products (and, therefore, unable to go more than a half-hour without a "fix")

- Have a seemingly-endless amount of advertising dollars, to convince you that, if you're not eating something every minute you're awake, you're not living "the good life"

- Have enough money to get government officials to "look the other way," while those food companies hawk their cookies and candy and donuts and ice cream, thereby turning this nation's biggest health crisis into a "Ho-hum" moment, as far as getting those government officials to **do** anything about it is concerned!

Or, to put it bluntly: Big Food has enough resources to get an endless number of people talking on its behalf (people we call "shills" or "lobbyists"), whereas there's **not enough money in the world** to get someone to put in a good word for cancer! So guess who comes out on the short end of **that** stick!

Like I say, you have to be amazed.

18

"Cheers!"

In *Walk Yourself Thin* and *Walk Yourself Fit*, we told you that real-world slimming—Thinwalking slimming, Fitwalking slimming—happens so gradually—at the rate of an ounce or two per day—that, if you expect to **see** any change in body size from one day to the next, all you'll be faced with is terminal disappointment.

Well, since then, we've come up with a really good way of illustrating this phenomenon:

Go to your kitchen cupboard—or your home bar—and pull out a shot glass (or, if you don't have a shot glass, then an egg cup, or one of your larger measuring spoons.) Place it on a counter. Look at it.

Got it?: that's what "an ounce or two" looks like.

Now, imagine that shot glass (or whatever) filled with body fat. Then imagine that amount of fat taken away, not just from **one tiny spot** on your body—where you probably **would** notice it—but from the **thousands of square inches** your body is made of: your arms, your legs, your stomach, your chest, etc.

You want to tell me the odds of **anyone** noticing **anything** leaving **anywhere**, when such a tiny amount is spread over such a vast area?

So, **don't** expect to notice it, because, if you do, you'll be forever disappointed.

And what happens when someone or something disappoints you?

Of course: if you're like most abusive eaters, who look to food for "comfort," "salving their wounds," etc., you go out and drown yourself in pancakes and Pop-tarts, thereby killing **whatever** size-loss program you were on.

Which is why we can't tell you enough: you're not here to **lose bodysize** (a.k.a., **weight**.) You're here to cure yourself of abusive eating; to take yourself to a whole new life, the life of a normal eater, since, once you've done that, the weight/bodysize will leave on its own.

Which means that, since you're not here to lose bodysize, it **won't matter** that you can't see any of it leaving on a day-to-day basis. Which means you **won't** be getting disappointed and **won't** be abandoning this program.

Which means this program will be taking you to the life you should have been living all along.

19

A Waste of Time

If there's one thing we know for sure it's that no oversized abusive eater has ever gone on a diet to lose weight.

"Excuse me?!"

I said—

"No, I heard what you said. But what you said is ridiculous! I mean, the whole **purpose** of a diet is to lose weight!"

Well, that may be true, but that's not the **reason** oversized people go on them.

"Then why else?"

This else:

1) One of the reasons oversized abusive eaters go on a diet is to "punish" themselves for being a "bad person."

Even though they may never say it out loud, down deep they know there's "something wrong" with stuffing your face all the time; that there's nothing "normal" about that, especially when years'-worth of stuffing has led to at least a year's-worth of food in storage—around their waist, hips, thighs, etc.—so how much additional "stuffing" could they possibly need?

Answer: none.

And what's the best way to "punish" yourself for stuffing your face all the time? Of course: stop stuffing your face altogether. In other words, go on a diet.

And what happens when you've punished yourself enough? Of course: you go off the diet.

And you have no problem with whatever weight your diet may have taken off you all going back on again, because **that's not why you went on the diet in the first place**, no matter how much it **seems** that's why you did.

2) The second reason oversized abusive eaters go on a diet is to show the world: "See: I'm doing something about my size. You said I should, and now I am. So, you'd better give me a ton of **kudos** for doing so."

And the world does, with people fawning all over you; praising you for finally taking your life in your own hands.

And what happens when you've shown "everybody" that you've finally decided to do something about your size by going on a diet?

Of course: you go **off** the diet. After all, you only went on it to **show** people something. And, once you've shown them **all**, what reason would you have for staying on it?

Answer: none. Which is why you have no problem going off it. Or with all the weight coming right back on that you've just taken off, since, again, losing weight was not why you went on the diet in the first place, so why would you object to that weight all coming back on again?

Answer: you wouldn't.

Look: no otherwise-healthy person in the history of the world has ever overeaten for the **purpose** of getting fat, any more than smokers smoke for the **purpose** of getting lung cancer, or drinkers drink for the **purpose** of turning their brains to soup and their liver and kidneys into shoe leather!

No, all those things—the fat, the lung cancer, the shoe leather, the soup—those are all **side** effects of abusers going after a **primary** effect: the "high" they get from their drug of choice, whether that drug is alcohol, nicotine, sugar or what-have-you.

So, since no one has ever eaten for the purpose of getting **fat**, why would anyone **change** the way they eat for the purpose of getting **thin**?

Answer: they wouldn't.

So that's why we can safely say: no oversized abusive eater has ever gone on a diet for the purpose of losing weight, no matter how much it looks like that's what they did.

And please keep in mind: when we say that no one has ever gone on a diet to lose weight, what we're saying is: no one has ever gone on a diet with an eye toward **permanent** weight loss.

As just mentioned: a diet is something you go **on**, the same way you get **on** an elevator, or a bus, or a plane. Meaning that, like that elevator, that bus, that plane, a diet is something you'll eventually go **off**, since no one I know has ever gotten **on** an elevator, a bus, or a plane without eventually getting **off**!

And what happens when you go off your diet?

Of course: you go back to eating the way you always have.

In other words, there's nothing "permanent" about a diet; at best, it's a temporary fix for a problem.

Which is why diets are a waste of time, as far as permanent weight loss is concerned, since whatever weight you lose on them will always go right back on again, since achieving permanent weight loss was not why you went on the diet in the first place; you only did it to punish yourself, or to show the world you were doing something about a problem, etc.

Which is why the only thing that will give you any **hope** for permanent weight loss/size loss is turning yourself into a normal eater.

Which, again, is why we're here.

20

The Non-diet Diet

At the start of the 21st century, the Subway chain of sandwich shops launched a campaign featuring a young man from Indianapolis, Jared Fogle (currently serving a 15-year sentence in federal prison for a variety of sex offenses), who had lost over 200 pounds in one year by switching from a zillion-calorie-a-day diet to eating a couple of Subway sandwiches every day, along with a small bag of chips and a diet soda.

Naturally, what the folks at Subway wanted you to believe is that it was their **sandwiches** that had led to Jared's weight loss—that there was something inherently **slimming** about their turkey club (Jared's lunch) and their veggie sub (Jared's dinner)—with the implication being that, if you ate those same sandwiches, you too would lose weight.

To which all we can say is: nice try, guys, but the plain truth is: it **wasn't** those sandwiches that were getting Jared thin; it was all the foods Jared was **no longer eating**—the food those sandwiches had **taken the place of**—that was doing the trick.

Why bring that up here?

Because, whether he realized it or not, what Jared had come up with was the best way to get unnecessary quantities of food in general—and of certain foods in particular—out of your life (and that we've used as the basis for our own program, especially our "addiction ladder" [Chapter 2]):

Using one food to get off of another

—in Jared's case: getting off of cheeseburgers and pizzas and pancakes and donuts by replacing them with a "**normal**" food that **no one** has a problem eating every day—things like turkey clubs and veggie subs—rather than what you find on your typical "diet," where they make you eat something that no one **wants** to eat, or can **stand** to eat, for more than a day or two—things like celery stalks and watercress sandwiches.

In other words, every day that Jared had a turkey club was a day he **didn't** have an extra-large pizza, a double Quarter Pounder, a half-dozen donuts, etc. And, as we've said, every day you do without something lessens that something's "pull" on you, until, after a week or two, that "pull" vanishes altogether. At which point, you're "cured" of that something.

In other words, Jared did the only thing you have to do, to turn yourself into a normal eater (and, in his case, lose 245 pounds): put **time** between you and your last pizza, your last Quarter Pounder, your last donut, etc.

So, do it. Pick out four or five non-addictive foods you enjoy eating—in my case, half a bagel and some eggs or a chunk of cheddar cheese for breakfast; a Swiss cheese sandwich for lunch; a salad or a pasta dish for dinner, with a piece of fruit for dessert—and eat those every day for the week or two it will take to get the foods they're replacing "out of your system."

Take it from us: you'll be glad you did!

21

Pants on Fire!

You're aware, of course, that there are people in this world who will say anything for money; will say anything their handlers tell them to say, as long as those handlers pay them enough.

Thus, the pathetic scene of people with a ton of fancy diplomas on the wall telling us:

- "There is, in fact, no scientific evidence that smoking causes lung cancer, or any other disease for that matter"—conveniently whistling right past the 40,000 studies that prove it does.

- "There are, in fact, alcoholics among us who can have a drink every now and then without falling off the wagon."

At which point, every alcoholic in the world points to the article and says, "See, I told you so," then rushes out and drowns himself in booze every day for the next five years!

- "There is no connection between obesity and disease. That's just something somebody made up, to scare us into losing all this excess bodysize, just because they find that bodysize disgusting to look at; because we 'muck up' their perfect little world!"

Which, of course, is total nonsense—obesity leads to an almost-un**countable** number of diseases—but that doesn't stop the abusive eater from wrapping his arms around the statement and racing off to the nearest soda fountain for a triple-dip banana split, since he now "knows" that banana split can't hurt him!

Why do these people do that? Why do these "authorities" lend their names and their prestige to such outlandish lies?

Because there are folks out there (who shall remain nameless, though, if we did name them, would have names like "food companies" and "tobacco companies" and "booze companies") that not only have a vested interest in you consuming their products, but have a vested interest in you believing those products will never **harm** you—and who've made enough money off you and others like you that they can now buy as many "authorities" as they like, to prove their point.

And, since the targets of all that nonsense are hopelessly addicted to those companies' products anyway, they jump for joy when they hear that those products are **totally harmless**, even if the "proof" that they're "totally harmless" has been pulled out of some authority's you-know-what!

Doesn't matter: those addicts' minds are now totally at ease. And stay at ease, till we bury them—10, 20, 30 years sooner than we should have had any need to—thanks to all those "totally harmless" cigarettes, beers, and hot fudge sundaes.

Why bring that up here?

Because if you're one of those people, living your life based on someone else's lie, then you yourself are living a lie, and you might want to wake up to that fact, and start listening to the people who **really** have your best interests at heart—me, for instance—and stop listening to people to whom you are

nothing more than a pocketbook, to be emptied as **often** and as **completely** as possible, and who will stop at nothing to keep that emptying going.

You with me?

WALKING

22

Before We Start Walking

Before we get into the walking part of this program—and because this world has gotten kind of "sue-happy" lately—we've got to tell you: if you're more than a few pounds oversized, you really should see a doctor first; make sure you're not looking at some sort of health risk here.

Of course, as we said in *Walk Yourself Thin* and *Walk Yourself Fit*, you have to be amazed:

Someone like Sara Lee or the Keebler Elves never have to tell you to "see a doctor" before you eat any of **their** stuff. And yet, their stuff tends to make people plus-sized, and plus-sized people tend to leave us a whole lot sooner than normal-sized people do, if I've been reading those insurance charts right.

And yet, those guys get **awards** for their stuff, while exercise pushers have to **tiptoe past courtrooms**!

Like I say: you have to be amazed!

So, do it; go see your doctor and get his "seal of approval."

Of course, while you're waiting to see him or her, you might want to strap on a pair of walking shoes and go slo-o-o-wly around the block a time or two.

Why?

Because then if Doc says you're **not** the one-in-a-million who shouldn't have, you'll be that many miles closer to a Beautiful New You!

23

Walking

So, time to go for a walk.

And, of course, when we say "walking," what we're talking about is "Thinwalking" or "Fitwalking," which is

> WALKING AS **FAST** AS YOU COMFORTABLY CAN FOR AS **LONG** AS YOU COMFORTABLY CAN.

What walking does is, it

• Uses up power molecules in your legs to fuel your walk, which molecules then have to be replaced, and it

• Breaks down some of the weaker muscle fibers in your legs, which then have to be rebuilt.

And where does your body get the raw materials to do all this molecule-replacing and muscle-rebuilding?

Of course: from your fat pads.

So, when you walk as fast as you comfortably can for as long as you comfortably can, you use up the most power molecules and break down the most muscle fibers you can. Which means your body will draw the most fat from your fat pads it possibly can. Which, when combined with your transition to normal eating, will get rid of your excess bodysize as fast as you possibly can.

Any questions?

24

The Value of Walking

When I give talks, I'll often ask the audience what they think the best thing about walking is. And what I usually get are:

"Walking burns calories, which makes losing bodysize that much easier."

"Walking makes you fitter."

"Walking can help ease the tensions of the day."

"Walking sets a good example for those around you."

—and on and on, with every reason as good as the ones before it.

However, as good as those reasons might be, there's one that people usually miss, and that might be the most valuable one of all:

The best thing about walking is that it gives you a **different way of looking at yourself**; lets you see yourself as something **other than an Eater**.

And why is that so important?

Because, as long as you see yourself as nothing but an Eater, what reason would you have for **not** eating?

However, the minute you see yourself, not only as an Eater, but as a Walker as well—even if only for a few minutes a day—then everything changes: now, instead of looking at a hot fudge sundae and saying, "Well, I have no reason not to eat it. I mean, it doesn't matter how much bodysize that sundae might wind up putting on me, since it's not exactly like I'm going to be **doing** anything with this body of mine," now you look at the sundae and say, "Y'know, I'd really love to have that sucker, but I did a wonderful three miles yesterday, and do I really want to **un**do all the good I did for myself, by giving in to my craving for that sundae, which I've already had a thousand of, these past few years, so do I really need another one?"

Once that thought process takes hold—that is, once you start seeing yourself as a Walker, as **well** as an Eater—your progression to normal eating—and all the wonders that come with it—is all but assured.

So, that's reason number one for turning yourself into a Walker: to see yourself as something other than an Eater, which will go a long way toward turning you into a **Normal** Eater, which is what we're all about.

And there's more:

We're all familiar with the saying, "Nothing succeeds like success." In other words, the more successes you have, the easier it is to have future ones.

Why is that so important?

Because the main "success" we're going for here is to have you turn yourself into a normal eater, which means exerting some control over yourself, over your eating, which can be difficult, given that we're fighting a lifetime of bad habits/addictions.

So, what would be nice would be for you to gain control over some aspect of your life that's **easy** to control, with the hope that success in that area will "spill over" and give you a greater chance of success in more **difficult** areas, like changing your eating.

And, if there's an aspect of our lives that's easier to control than walking—"Put Foot A in front of Foot B; repeat with Foot B"—I'm at a loss to know what it might be!

So, that's another major reason for walking: because it will give you a "success" in one area that should make it easier to achieve success in others.

Again: "Nothing succeeds like success."

And one more reason becoming a Walker is so valuable:

When you're strictly an Eater, we all know where every extra French fry or piece of bread you eat will eventually wind up. Which is why, when you decide to lose a little bodysize/weight, those French fries and extra pieces of bread suddenly become "forbidden fruit."

However, the minute you add **walking** to your eating life, that all changes: now, instead of being "afraid" of those French fries, those pieces of bread, you have "no problem" eating them.

Why?

Because you know that within minutes or hours you'll be **walking them all off**, meaning they **won't** be winding up you-know-where, so what's to be afraid of?!

Meaning you can **enjoy** a French fry or two or an extra piece of bread every now and then, the way every normal eater does!

I'm sure you can add several more great reasons for becoming a walker to that list, so feel free to do so.

For now, though, those three should get you started.

25

Lipo

Whether or not they'll admit it, it's every oversized person's dream to go to sleep fat and wake up thin.

Until recently, of course, that's all it could be: a dream.

But not anymore.

Oh no. Now, thanks to something called "liposuction," you **can** do exactly that: go to sleep fat and wake up thin.

Which is fine, except: like any surgical procedure, this one is not without its downsides:

1) First of all, when you add in all the costs—the surgery, the anesthesia, the operating room staff, the hospitalization, etc.—the whole thing can get rather expensive: something on the order of $10,000, if you're going to be doing more than one body area at a time, which you usually are.

2) Since liposuction is an **elective** procedure—that is, something you **choose** to do, rather than something you **have** to do—most insurance plans won't cover it, so guess who winds up footing the bill?

3) You don't **really** "go to sleep fat and wake up thin." As it happens, it usually takes **several months** for your new shape to "kick in."

So, if you really **were** thinking of liposuction as an overnight fix, you might not be all that happy with the way you look when you wake up.

4) As with any procedure where they have to put to sleep, the risk of never waking up again is always there—though, to be perfectly honest, that risk is so small nowadays as to be virtually non-existent. However, it's not **totally** non-existent, so you should be aware of it.

5) Again, as with most surgeries, this one is not without post-surgical pain—and usually lots of it.

Yes, you can take all manner of pills to alleviate the pain. However, as this nation's opiod crisis has shown us, there's "no free lunch" there either.

So, yes: it's now possible to "go to sleep fat and wake up thin"—as long as you don't mind all the downsides that come with it.

Of course, it's not really necessary to go through all the expense, risk, and pain of actual liposuction to get every drop of fat sucked off you. Oh no: the fact is, you can get all the liposuction you want, and without getting anywhere near a surgeon or putting out a penny.

How so?

Well, what **is** liposuction?

Of course: a procedure where a machine sucks fat from wherever it's stored.

Usually, that machine is in a surgeon's office, or an operating room. But it doesn't have to be.

No: as luck would have it, you already **own** a liposuction machine—**two** of them, in fact.

That's right.

They're those things dangling from your hips—commonly known as "leg muscles"—and, when you turn **those** liposuction machines on—by going out for a walk—they do exactly what an **actual** liposuction machine does: they suck fat from wherever it's stored and get rid of it—in this case, not throwing it in the trash, the way a surgeon would, but, instead, using it to replace the power molecules your walk has used up, and to rebuild the muscles your walk has torn down.

True, your built-in liposuction machines may not suck up as much fat per day as your **doctor's** machine would, but who cares: they **do suck up fat**, and without any of the cost, pain, risk, etc., of **actual** liposuction.

So, the next time you go out for a Thinwalk or a Fitwalk, you might want to keep that in mind: that every step you take sucks a little bit of fat from wherever it's stored: your legs, your waist, your hips, your thighs, etc.; meaning that, the more steps you take, the more fat gets sucked up, until the inevitable day that it's **all** been sucked up.

Of course, no matter which liposuction machine we're talking about—your doctor's or the ones you've been carrying around since birth—neither is worth a damn if you **never turn it on**!

26

Greatest Feeling

Want to know the greatest feeling in the world (no: **aside** from that!)?

The greatest feeling in the world is: going to bed, hours after you've finished a one-, two-, or three-mile walk, and having it feel like a million flashbulbs are going off, one after the other, up and down your legs!

And why is that the greatest feeling in the world?

Because it's **proof-positive** that your **walking is working**; that it's using up power molecules, which have to be replaced, and tearing down muscle fibers, which have to be rebuilt.

Which is exactly what every one of those "flashbulbs" signifies: a power molecule being replaced or a muscle fiber being rebuilt.

And, if that's not the greatest feeling in the world—having **physical evidence** that what we said would happen is, in fact, happening—then I don't know what would be.

And want to know the **second**-greatest feeling in the world?: waking up six or eight hours later with those "flashbulbs" **still going off**!

To which, all we can say is: enjoy the show!

27

The Golden Itch

Anyone who's taken a first-aid class knows what happens when you apply a tourniquet to someone's arm, to stop blood from flowing into it, and then release the tourniquet a minute or two later: blood rushing back into an area where it hasn't been for a while makes the arm **itch like crazy**!

So what?

So, even though blood has obviously been flowing into and out of your fat pads—else they, and you, would have been dead a long time ago—the fact is, not a whole **lot** of blood has been flowing into and out of them; in fact, only enough to drop off, or pick up, a tiny bit of fat every now and then.

So what?

So, once you start Thinwalking or Fitwalking, and get to walking fast enough and far enough for your walking to be classed as "exercise"—or once you're down to eating next-to-nothing every day, the way normal eaters eat—there will come a time when the food in your gut—the food you've eaten—is not enough to satisfy your body's energy needs. Which means your body is going to have to look elsewhere to satisfy those needs.

Where else?

Of course: your fat pads.

So, there you'll be, out walking to "beat the band"—or reveling in the glow of finally eating like a normal human being—when suddenly, the skin over your fat pads—usually your belly, but it could be anywhere—starts to **itch like crazy**!

At which point you'll stop—literally or figuratively—and say to yourself: "Wait a minute! What's going on here? I took a shower this morning, so I can't be itching because I'm 'dirty.' And I don't have hives, so that can't be the answer. So, what's going on here?"

What's going on is exactly what went on in that first-aid class: blood suddenly rushing into an area where it hasn't been for awhile—or at least not in any great quantity—as it looks for food it couldn't find anywhere else.

And why do we refer to this itch as "golden"?

Easy: because it shows that **the program is working**; that all that walking—or normal eating—is doing what it's supposed to do: getting your body to start using **stored** energy for a change, rather than energy from the "usual suspect:" your gut. Meaning those storage "depots"—your fat pads—will soon start shrinking, which is exactly why we're here.

Will this happen to everybody?

We don't know.

But if it happens to you, it should take a bulldozer to wipe the smile off your face.

It did ours!

28

"Just Do It!"

A while back, a newspaper reporter went out to interview the late fitness guru Jack LaLanne (1914-2011).

Noting LaLanne's incredible physique, the reporter said, "Man, you must love to exercise!"

To which LaLanne replied, "Are you kidding: I **hate** to exercise—" which made the reporter do a double-take, not believing what he was hearing, until he saw the smile creep up on LaLanne's face, "—but I **love the results**!"

You get it? Of **course** exercise can be a pain in the ass. Much easier to just sit on the couch and toss bonbons down your throat all day!

Except…

As we've said elsewhere, there **will be a tomorrow**; there always is.

So, you have to ask yourself: "What do I want that tomorrow to look like?

"If I stick with the bonbons, they're sure-as-hell gonna 'stick' with me!

"However, if I take a minute or two every day to use something other than my chewing muscles—say, my leg muscles, by taking a walk, or my arm muscles, by doing a few curls with some free weights while I watch TV—mightn't that do more for my tomorrow—make it a little better-looking and a little better-feeling—than just sticking to my daily bonbon routine?"

Answer: yes, it will.

So, as the Nike ad used to tell us: "Just do it!" Stop finding reasons for **not** taking a walk and just **take** one.

And don't worry about walking "a mile." Or "two miles." Or "five."

Again: "A journey of a thousand miles begins with a single step." In other words, it doesn't matter how many miles you were **planning** on doing: until you take that first step, **no** mileage is possible!

So, do it; take that first step.

And maybe, by doing so, you'll discover what every other Thinwalker and Fitwalker has: that taking that first step makes the second one a whole lot easier!

And the third.

And the fourth.

-
-
-
-

29

"That's a Wrap!"

So there you have it—the whole program—which asks only this of you:

1) That you take as much time as you need, to convince yourself that, if you're more than a few pounds oversized, then virtually all the hunger pangs you feel in the course of a day are phony; that they have absolutely nothing to do with a real need for food, your body's need for food, no matter how real they might feel; that all they are is something cooked up by your Subconscious Mind to get you doing the same things today that you did yesterday, thinking that's what you need to do to survive, even though you don't.

Which means there's no reason to **respond** to those hunger pangs, no reason to **"feed"** them, or, if you do feed them, then to feed them only as much real food as it would take to make them go away.

2) That you realize that by not feeding those phony hunger pangs—or feeding them as little as it would take to make them go away—they will eventually stop bothering you.

At which point, you'll be "cured" of those hunger pangs; which means you'll be cured of abusive eating; which means that whatever excess bodysize you've been carrying around will soon be gone, because there will be nothing left to sustain it.

3) That you start walking a little faster and a little farther each day—naturally, after getting your doctor's OK to do so—so that, if an extra calorie or two does slip past your watchful eye, it will wind up getting **burned**—in the "metabolic furnaces" known as your leg muscles—rather than **stored**, in you-know-what.

And that's it! That's all you have to do, to take yourself to the life you should have been living all along, and would have been living, if someone hadn't given you a different one, long before you were old enough or smart enough to know what they were doing to you. In other words, the life that normal eaters live every day, and that you have no reason not to.

The Log

What follows is a Weekly Log, to help you keep track of what your walking program is doing for you.

We've tried to make it as easy as possible for you to keep this Log—for example, using lots of check marks, rather than asking you to write a term paper every few days!

Oh, and if you'd rather not write in the book—if, for example, you don't own it—just photocopy as many Log pages as you'd like and create your **own** Log book.

As you'll notice, our main concern here is with "subjective" results—you being the "subject"—things like how you feel overall; how your legs feel; how easy your walk was; etc.

Naturally, we've also allocated space for "objective" results—that is, things measured by some physical object, like a stopwatch, pedometer, etc. However, we consider those far less important than knowing the way you're changing "personally" from one week to the next. Which is why we've placed those objective measurements at the **bottom** of each Log page, and labeled them "Optional."

Anyway, have fun with this Log, and feel free to let us know how you like it.

126 *Enough is Enough!*

Weekly Log

Week No.:_____ Date:_____ Approx. Time of Day: _____ to _____

About how far did you walk today?_____

How does that distance compare with how far you walked a week ago?
- ❏ Much farther
- ❏ A little farther
- ❏ About the same
- ❏ Not as far

About how fast did you walk today (on average?)
- ❏ Over 30 min./mile
- ❏ 25-30 min./mile
- ❏ 20-25 min./mile
- ❏ 17-19 min./mile
- ❏ 15-16 min./mile
- ❏ 13-14 min./mile
- ❏ 10-12 min./mile
- ❏ Less than 10

How does this compare with how fast you walked a week ago?
- ❏ Much faster
- ❏ A little faster
- ❏ About the same
- ❏ A little slower

How did your leg muscles feel at the start of your walk?
- ❏ Loose and "fluid"
- ❏ About "normal"
- ❏ Somewhat "stiff"
- ❏ Very "stiff"
- ❏ Painful
- ❏ "Tired" or "Empty"

How did your leg muscles feel at the mid-point of your walk?
- ❏ Loose and "fluid"
- ❏ About "normal"
- ❏ Somewhat "stiff"
- ❏ Very "stiff"
- ❏ Painful
- ❏ "Tired" or "Empty"

How did your leg muscles feel at the end of your walk?
- ❏ Loose and "fluid"
- ❏ About "normal"
- ❏ Somewhat "stiff"
- ❏ Very "stiff"
- ❏ Painful
- ❏ "Tired" or "Empty"

How would you describe the way you were breathing at the "height" of your walk?
- ❏ With great difficulty
- ❏ With some difficulty
- ❏ "Normally"
- ❏ Very easily

What clothing size were you able to fit into this morning?
- ❏ Slack size:
- ❏ Dress size (if applicable):

How would you describe the "fit?"
- ❏ Very tight
- ❏ Somewhat tight
- ❏ "Just right"
- ❏ A bit loose
- ❏ Very loose
- ❏ Walked right out of them!

Overall Impressions and Comments on Your Progress:

Optional Walking Log: Lap Length: _____

Lap No.	1	2	3	4	5	6	7	8
Lap Time								
Cum. Time								

Comments:

Weekly Log

Week No.:_____ Date: _____ Approx. Time of Day: _____ to _____

About how far did you walk today?_____

How does that distance compare with how far you walked a week ago?
- ❏ Much farther
- ❏ A little farther
- ❏ About the same
- ❏ Not as far

About how fast did you walk today (on average?)
- ❏ Over 30 min./mile
- ❏ 20-25 min./mile
- ❏ 15-16 min./mile
- ❏ 10-12 min./mile
- ❏ 25-30 min./mile
- ❏ 17-19 min./mile
- ❏ 13-14 min./mile
- ❏ Less than 10

How does this compare with how fast you walked a week ago?
- ❏ Much faster
- ❏ A little faster
- ❏ About the same
- ❏ A little slower

How did your leg muscles feel at the start of your walk?
- ❏ Loose and "fluid"
- ❏ About "normal"
- ❏ Somewhat "stiff"
- ❏ Very "stiff"
- ❏ Painful
- ❏ "Tired" or "Empty"

How did your leg muscles feel at the mid-point of your walk?
- ❏ Loose and "fluid"
- ❏ About "normal"
- ❏ Somewhat "stiff"
- ❏ Very "stiff"
- ❏ Painful
- ❏ "Tired" or "Empty"

How did your leg muscles feel at the end of your walk?
- ❏ Loose and "fluid"
- ❏ About "normal"
- ❏ Somewhat "stiff"
- ❏ Very "stiff"
- ❏ Painful
- ❏ "Tired" or "Empty"

How would you describe the way you were breathing at the "height" of your walk?
- ❏ With great difficulty
- ❏ With some difficulty
- ❏ "Normally"
- ❏ Very easily

What clothing size were you able to fit into this morning?
- ❏ Slack size:
- ❏ Dress size (if applicable):

How would you describe the "fit?"
- ❏ Very tight
- ❏ Somewhat tight
- ❏ "Just right"
- ❏ A bit loose
- ❏ Very loose
- ❏ Walked right out of them!

Overall Impressions and Comments on Your Progress:

Optional Walking Log: Lap Length: _____

Lap No.	1	2	3	4	5	6	7	8
Lap Time								
Cum. Time								

Comments:

128 *Enough is Enough!*

Weekly Log

Week No.:_____ Date: _____ Approx. Time of Day: _____ to _____

About how far did you walk today?_____

How does that distance compare with how far you walked a week ago?
- ❏ Much farther
- ❏ A little farther
- ❏ About the same
- ❏ Not as far

About how fast did you walk today (on average?)
- ❏ Over 30 min./mile
- ❏ 25-30 min./mile
- ❏ 20-25 min./mile
- ❏ 17-19 min./mile
- ❏ 15-16 min./mile
- ❏ 13-14 min./mile
- ❏ 10-12 min./mile
- ❏ Less than 10

How does this compare with how fast you walked a week ago?
- ❏ Much faster
- ❏ A little faster
- ❏ About the same
- ❏ A little slower

How did your leg muscles feel at the start of your walk?
- ❏ Loose and "fluid"
- ❏ About "normal"
- ❏ Somewhat "stiff"
- ❏ Very "stiff"
- ❏ Painful
- ❏ "Tired" or "Empty"

How did your leg muscles feel at the mid-point of your walk?
- ❏ Loose and "fluid"
- ❏ About "normal"
- ❏ Somewhat "stiff"
- ❏ Very "stiff"
- ❏ Painful
- ❏ "Tired" or "Empty"

How did your leg muscles feel at the end of your walk?
- ❏ Loose and "fluid"
- ❏ About "normal"
- ❏ Somewhat "stiff"
- ❏ Very "stiff"
- ❏ Painful
- ❏ "Tired" or "Empty"

How would you describe the way you were breathing at the "height" of your walk?
- ❏ With great difficulty
- ❏ With some difficulty
- ❏ "Normally"
- ❏ Very easily

What clothing size were you able to fit into this morning?
- ❏ Slack size:
- ❏ Dress size (if applicable):

How would you describe the "fit?"
- ❏ Very tight
- ❏ Somewhat tight
- ❏ "Just right"
- ❏ A bit loose
- ❏ Very loose
- ❏ Walked right out of them!

Overall Impressions and Comments on Your Progress:

Optional Walking Log: Lap Length: _____

Lap No.	1	2	3	4	5	6	7	8
Lap Time								
Cum. Time								

Comments:

Weekly Log

Week No.:_____ Date: _____ Approx. Time of Day: _____ to _____

About how far did you walk today?_____

How does that distance compare with how far you walked a week ago?
        ❏ Much farther   ❏ About the same
        ❏ A little farther   ❏ Not as far

About how fast did you walk today (on average?)
❏ Over 30 min./mile   ❏ 20-25 min./mile   ❏ 15-16 min./mile   ❏ 10-12 min./mile
❏ 25-30 min./mile   ❏ 17-19 min./mile   ❏ 13-14 min./mile   ❏ Less than 10

How does this compare with how fast you walked a week ago?
        ❏ Much faster   ❏ About the same
        ❏ A little faster   ❏ A little slower

How did your leg muscles feel at the start of your walk?
    ❏ Loose and "fluid"   ❏ Somewhat "stiff"   ❏ Painful
    ❏ About "normal"   ❏ Very "stiff"   ❏ "Tired" or "Empty"

How did your leg muscles feel at the mid-point of your walk?
    ❏ Loose and "fluid"   ❏ Somewhat "stiff"   ❏ Painful
    ❏ About "normal"   ❏ Very "stiff"   ❏ "Tired" or "Empty"

How did your leg muscles feel at the end of your walk?
    ❏ Loose and "fluid"   ❏ Somewhat "stiff"   ❏ Painful
    ❏ About "normal"   ❏ Very "stiff"   ❏ "Tired" or "Empty"

How would you describe the way you were breathing at the "height" of your walk?
        ❏ With great difficulty   ❏ "Normally"
        ❏ With some difficulty   ❏ Very easily

What clothing size were you able to fit into this morning?
        ❏ Slack size:
        ❏ Dress size (if applicable):

How would you describe the "fit?"
    ❏ Very tight   ❏ "Just right"   ❏ Very loose
    ❏ Somewhat tight   ❏ A bit loose   ❏ Walked right out of them!

Overall Impressions and Comments on Your Progress:

Optional Walking Log: Lap Length: _____

Lap No.	1	2	3	4	5	6	7	8
Lap Time								
Cum. Time								

Comments:

Weekly Log

Week No.:_____ Date: _____ Approx. Time of Day: _____ to _____

About how far did you walk today?_____

How does that distance compare with how far you walked a week ago?
       ❑ Much farther   ❑ About the same
       ❑ A little farther   ❑ Not as far

About how fast did you walk today (on average?)
❑ Over 30 min./mile   ❑ 20-25 min./mile   ❑ 15-16 min./mile   ❑ 10-12 min./mile
❑ 25-30 min./mile   ❑ 17-19 min./mile   ❑ 13-14 min./mile   ❑ Less than 10

How does this compare with how fast you walked a week ago?
       ❑ Much faster   ❑ About the same
       ❑ A little faster   ❑ A little slower

How did your leg muscles feel at the start of your walk?
    ❑ Loose and "fluid"   ❑ Somewhat "stiff"   ❑ Painful
    ❑ About "normal"   ❑ Very "stiff"   ❑ "Tired" or "Empty"

How did your leg muscles feel at the mid-point of your walk?
    ❑ Loose and "fluid"   ❑ Somewhat "stiff"   ❑ Painful
    ❑ About "normal"   ❑ Very "stiff"   ❑ "Tired" or "Empty"

How did your leg muscles feel at the end of your walk?
    ❑ Loose and "fluid"   ❑ Somewhat "stiff"   ❑ Painful
    ❑ About "normal"   ❑ Very "stiff"   ❑ "Tired" or "Empty"

How would you describe the way you were breathing at the "height" of your walk?
        ❑ With great difficulty   ❑ "Normally"
        ❑ With some difficulty   ❑ Very easily

What clothing size were you able to fit into this morning?
        ❑ Slack size:
        ❑ Dress size (if applicable):

How would you describe the "fit?"
    ❑ Very tight   ❑ "Just right"   ❑ Very loose
    ❑ Somewhat tight   ❑ A bit loose   ❑ Walked right out of them!

Overall Impressions and Comments on Your Progress:

Optional Walking Log: Lap Length: _____

Lap No.	1	2	3	4	5	6	7	8
Lap Time								
Cum. Time								

Comments:

Weekly Log

Week No.:_____ Date: _____ Approx. Time of Day: _____ to _____

About how far did you walk today?_____

How does that distance compare with how far you walked a week ago?
- ❏ Much farther
- ❏ A little farther
- ❏ About the same
- ❏ Not as far

About how fast did you walk today (on average?)
- ❏ Over 30 min./mile
- ❏ 25-30 min./mile
- ❏ 20-25 min./mile
- ❏ 17-19 min./mile
- ❏ 15-16 min./mile
- ❏ 13-14 min./mile
- ❏ 10-12 min./mile
- ❏ Less than 10

How does this compare with how fast you walked a week ago?
- ❏ Much faster
- ❏ A little faster
- ❏ About the same
- ❏ A little slower

How did your leg muscles feel at the start of your walk?
- ❏ Loose and "fluid"
- ❏ About "normal"
- ❏ Somewhat "stiff"
- ❏ Very "stiff"
- ❏ Painful
- ❏ "Tired" or "Empty"

How did your leg muscles feel at the mid-point of your walk?
- ❏ Loose and "fluid"
- ❏ About "normal"
- ❏ Somewhat "stiff"
- ❏ Very "stiff"
- ❏ Painful
- ❏ "Tired" or "Empty"

How did your leg muscles feel at the end of your walk?
- ❏ Loose and "fluid"
- ❏ About "normal"
- ❏ Somewhat "stiff"
- ❏ Very "stiff"
- ❏ Painful
- ❏ "Tired" or "Empty"

How would you describe the way you were breathing at the "height" of your walk?
- ❏ With great difficulty
- ❏ With some difficulty
- ❏ "Normally"
- ❏ Very easily

What clothing size were you able to fit into this morning?
- ❏ Slack size:
- ❏ Dress size (if applicable):

How would you describe the "fit?"
- ❏ Very tight
- ❏ Somewhat tight
- ❏ "Just right"
- ❏ A bit loose
- ❏ Very loose
- ❏ Walked right out of them!

Overall Impressions and Comments on Your Progress:

Optional Walking Log: Lap Length: _____

Lap No.	1	2	3	4	5	6	7	8
Lap Time								
Cum. Time								

Comments:

Weekly Log

Week No.:_____ Date: _____ Approx. Time of Day: _____ to _____

About how far did you walk today?_____

How does that distance compare with how far you walked a week ago?
- ❏ Much farther
- ❏ A little farther
- ❏ About the same
- ❏ Not as far

About how fast did you walk today (on average?)
- ❏ Over 30 min./mile
- ❏ 25-30 min./mile
- ❏ 20-25 min./mile
- ❏ 17-19 min./mile
- ❏ 15-16 min./mile
- ❏ 13-14 min./mile
- ❏ 10-12 min./mile
- ❏ Less than 10

How does this compare with how fast you walked a week ago?
- ❏ Much faster
- ❏ A little faster
- ❏ About the same
- ❏ A little slower

How did your leg muscles feel at the start of your walk?
- ❏ Loose and "fluid"
- ❏ About "normal"
- ❏ Somewhat "stiff"
- ❏ Very "stiff"
- ❏ Painful
- ❏ "Tired" or "Empty"

How did your leg muscles feel at the mid-point of your walk?
- ❏ Loose and "fluid"
- ❏ About "normal"
- ❏ Somewhat "stiff"
- ❏ Very "stiff"
- ❏ Painful
- ❏ "Tired" or "Empty"

How did your leg muscles feel at the end of your walk?
- ❏ Loose and "fluid"
- ❏ About "normal"
- ❏ Somewhat "stiff"
- ❏ Very "stiff"
- ❏ Painful
- ❏ "Tired" or "Empty"

How would you describe the way you were breathing at the "height" of your walk?
- ❏ With great difficulty
- ❏ With some difficulty
- ❏ "Normally"
- ❏ Very easily

What clothing size were you able to fit into this morning?
- ❏ Slack size:
- ❏ Dress size (if applicable):

How would you describe the "fit?"
- ❏ Very tight
- ❏ Somewhat tight
- ❏ "Just right"
- ❏ A bit loose
- ❏ Very loose
- ❏ Walked right out of them!

Overall Impressions and Comments on Your Progress:

Optional Walking Log: Lap Length: _____

Lap No.	1	2	3	4	5	6	7	8
Lap Time								
Cum. Time								

Comments:

Weekly Log

Week No.:_____ Date: _____ Approx. Time of Day: _____ to _____

About how far did you walk today?_____

How does that distance compare with how far you walked a week ago?
- ❏ Much farther
- ❏ A little farther
- ❏ About the same
- ❏ Not as far

About how fast did you walk today (on average?)
- ❏ Over 30 min./mile
- ❏ 20-25 min./mile
- ❏ 15-16 min./mile
- ❏ 10-12 min./mile
- ❏ 25-30 min./mile
- ❏ 17-19 min./mile
- ❏ 13-14 min./mile
- ❏ Less than 10

How does this compare with how fast you walked a week ago?
- ❏ Much faster
- ❏ A little faster
- ❏ About the same
- ❏ A little slower

How did your leg muscles feel at the start of your walk?
- ❏ Loose and "fluid"
- ❏ About "normal"
- ❏ Somewhat "stiff"
- ❏ Very "stiff"
- ❏ Painful
- ❏ "Tired" or "Empty"

How did your leg muscles feel at the mid-point of your walk?
- ❏ Loose and "fluid"
- ❏ About "normal"
- ❏ Somewhat "stiff"
- ❏ Very "stiff"
- ❏ Painful
- ❏ "Tired" or "Empty"

How did your leg muscles feel at the end of your walk?
- ❏ Loose and "fluid"
- ❏ About "normal"
- ❏ Somewhat "stiff"
- ❏ Very "stiff"
- ❏ Painful
- ❏ "Tired" or "Empty"

How would you describe the way you were breathing at the "height" of your walk?
- ❏ With great difficulty
- ❏ With some difficulty
- ❏ "Normally"
- ❏ Very easily

What clothing size were you able to fit into this morning?
- ❏ Slack size:
- ❏ Dress size (if applicable):

How would you describe the "fit?"
- ❏ Very tight
- ❏ Somewhat tight
- ❏ "Just right"
- ❏ A bit loose
- ❏ Very loose
- ❏ Walked right out of them!

Overall Impressions and Comments on Your Progress:

Optional Walking Log: Lap Length: _____

Lap No.	1	2	3	4	5	6	7	8
Lap Time								
Cum. Time								

Comments:

Weekly Log

Week No.:_____ Date: _____ Approx. Time of Day: _____ to _____

About how far did you walk today?_____

How does that distance compare with how far you walked a week ago?
         ❏ Much farther   ❏ About the same
         ❏ A little farther   ❏ Not as far

About how fast did you walk today (on average?)
❏ Over 30 min./mile   ❏ 20-25 min./mile   ❏ 15-16 min./mile   ❏ 10-12 min./mile
❏ 25-30 min./mile   ❏ 17-19 min./mile   ❏ 13-14 min./mile   ❏ Less than 10

How does this compare with how fast you walked a week ago?
         ❏ Much faster   ❏ About the same
         ❏ A little faster   ❏ A little slower

How did your leg muscles feel at the start of your walk?
     ❏ Loose and "fluid"   ❏ Somewhat "stiff"   ❏ Painful
     ❏ About "normal"   ❏ Very "stiff"   ❏ "Tired" or "Empty"

How did your leg muscles feel at the mid-point of your walk?
     ❏ Loose and "fluid"   ❏ Somewhat "stiff"   ❏ Painful
     ❏ About "normal"   ❏ Very "stiff"   ❏ "Tired" or "Empty"

How did your leg muscles feel at the end of your walk?
     ❏ Loose and "fluid"   ❏ Somewhat "stiff"   ❏ Painful
     ❏ About "normal"   ❏ Very "stiff"   ❏ "Tired" or "Empty"

How would you describe the way you were breathing at the "height" of your walk?
         ❏ With great difficulty   ❏ "Normally"
         ❏ With some difficulty   ❏ Very easily

What clothing size were you able to fit into this morning?
         ❏ Slack size:
         ❏ Dress size (if applicable):

How would you describe the "fit?"
     ❏ Very tight   ❏ "Just right"   ❏ Very loose
     ❏ Somewhat tight   ❏ A bit loose   ❏ Walked right out of them!

Overall Impressions and Comments on Your Progress:

Optional Walking Log: Lap Length: _____

Lap No.	1	2	3	4	5	6	7	8
Lap Time								
Cum. Time								

Comments:

Weekly Log

Week No.:_____ Date: _____ Approx. Time of Day: _____ to _____

About how far did you walk today?_____

How does that distance compare with how far you walked a week ago?
- ❏ Much farther
- ❏ A little farther
- ❏ About the same
- ❏ Not as far

About how fast did you walk today (on average?)
- ❏ Over 30 min./mile
- ❏ 25-30 min./mile
- ❏ 20-25 min./mile
- ❏ 17-19 min./mile
- ❏ 15-16 min./mile
- ❏ 13-14 min./mile
- ❏ 10-12 min./mile
- ❏ Less than 10

How does this compare with how fast you walked a week ago?
- ❏ Much faster
- ❏ A little faster
- ❏ About the same
- ❏ A little slower

How did your leg muscles feel at the start of your walk?
- ❏ Loose and "fluid"
- ❏ About "normal"
- ❏ Somewhat "stiff"
- ❏ Very "stiff"
- ❏ Painful
- ❏ "Tired" or "Empty"

How did your leg muscles feel at the mid-point of your walk?
- ❏ Loose and "fluid"
- ❏ About "normal"
- ❏ Somewhat "stiff"
- ❏ Very "stiff"
- ❏ Painful
- ❏ "Tired" or "Empty"

How did your leg muscles feel at the end of your walk?
- ❏ Loose and "fluid"
- ❏ About "normal"
- ❏ Somewhat "stiff"
- ❏ Very "stiff"
- ❏ Painful
- ❏ "Tired" or "Empty"

How would you describe the way you were breathing at the "height" of your walk?
- ❏ With great difficulty
- ❏ With some difficulty
- ❏ "Normally"
- ❏ Very easily

What clothing size were you able to fit into this morning?
- ❏ Slack size:
- ❏ Dress size (if applicable):

How would you describe the "fit?"
- ❏ Very tight
- ❏ Somewhat tight
- ❏ "Just right"
- ❏ A bit loose
- ❏ Very loose
- ❏ Walked right out of them!

Overall Impressions and Comments on Your Progress:

Optional Walking Log: Lap Length: _____

Lap No.	1	2	3	4	5	6	7	8
Lap Time								
Cum. Time								

Comments:

Weekly Log

Week No.:_____ Date: _____ Approx. Time of Day: _____ to _____

About how far did you walk today?_____

How does that distance compare with how far you walked a week ago?
- ❏ Much farther
- ❏ A little farther
- ❏ About the same
- ❏ Not as far

About how fast did you walk today (on average?)
- ❏ Over 30 min./mile
- ❏ 25-30 min./mile
- ❏ 20-25 min./mile
- ❏ 17-19 min./mile
- ❏ 15-16 min./mile
- ❏ 13-14 min./mile
- ❏ 10-12 min./mile
- ❏ Less than 10

How does this compare with how fast you walked a week ago?
- ❏ Much faster
- ❏ A little faster
- ❏ About the same
- ❏ A little slower

How did your leg muscles feel at the start of your walk?
- ❏ Loose and "fluid"
- ❏ About "normal"
- ❏ Somewhat "stiff"
- ❏ Very "stiff"
- ❏ Painful
- ❏ "Tired" or "Empty"

How did your leg muscles feel at the mid-point of your walk?
- ❏ Loose and "fluid"
- ❏ About "normal"
- ❏ Somewhat "stiff"
- ❏ Very "stiff"
- ❏ Painful
- ❏ "Tired" or "Empty"

How did your leg muscles feel at the end of your walk?
- ❏ Loose and "fluid"
- ❏ About "normal"
- ❏ Somewhat "stiff"
- ❏ Very "stiff"
- ❏ Painful
- ❏ "Tired" or "Empty"

How would you describe the way you were breathing at the "height" of your walk?
- ❏ With great difficulty
- ❏ With some difficulty
- ❏ "Normally"
- ❏ Very easily

What clothing size were you able to fit into this morning?
- ❏ Slack size:
- ❏ Dress size (if applicable):

How would you describe the "fit?"
- ❏ Very tight
- ❏ Somewhat tight
- ❏ "Just right"
- ❏ A bit loose
- ❏ Very loose
- ❏ Walked right out of them!

Overall Impressions and Comments on Your Progress:

Optional Walking Log: Lap Length: _____

Lap No.	1	2	3	4	5	6	7	8
Lap Time								
Cum. Time								

Comments:

Weekly Log

Week No.:_____ Date: _____ Approx. Time of Day: _____ to _____

About how far did you walk today?_____

How does that distance compare with how far you walked a week ago?
- ❏ Much farther
- ❏ A little farther
- ❏ About the same
- ❏ Not as far

About how fast did you walk today (on average?)
- ❏ Over 30 min./mile
- ❏ 25-30 min./mile
- ❏ 20-25 min./mile
- ❏ 17-19 min./mile
- ❏ 15-16 min./mile
- ❏ 13-14 min./mile
- ❏ 10-12 min./mile
- ❏ Less than 10

How does this compare with how fast you walked a week ago?
- ❏ Much faster
- ❏ A little faster
- ❏ About the same
- ❏ A little slower

How did your leg muscles feel at the start of your walk?
- ❏ Loose and "fluid"
- ❏ About "normal"
- ❏ Somewhat "stiff"
- ❏ Very "stiff"
- ❏ Painful
- ❏ "Tired" or "Empty"

How did your leg muscles feel at the mid-point of your walk?
- ❏ Loose and "fluid"
- ❏ About "normal"
- ❏ Somewhat "stiff"
- ❏ Very "stiff"
- ❏ Painful
- ❏ "Tired" or "Empty"

How did your leg muscles feel at the end of your walk?
- ❏ Loose and "fluid"
- ❏ About "normal"
- ❏ Somewhat "stiff"
- ❏ Very "stiff"
- ❏ Painful
- ❏ "Tired" or "Empty"

How would you describe the way you were breathing at the "height" of your walk?
- ❏ With great difficulty
- ❏ With some difficulty
- ❏ "Normally"
- ❏ Very easily

What clothing size were you able to fit into this morning?
- ❏ Slack size:
- ❏ Dress size (if applicable):

How would you describe the "fit?"
- ❏ Very tight
- ❏ Somewhat tight
- ❏ "Just right"
- ❏ A bit loose
- ❏ Very loose
- ❏ Walked right out of them!

Overall Impressions and Comments on Your Progress:

Optional Walking Log: Lap Length: _____

Lap No.	1	2	3	4	5	6	7	8
Lap Time								
Cum. Time								

Comments:

Appendix

Like it says on the cover, this book contains the cure. For a disease.

At first, we weren't all that crazy about calling this thing a "disease;" after all, who likes to think of themselves as "sick"?

Until, one day, it dawned on us that what we're talking about here disables and kills more Americans before their time than a host of other diseases **combined**—mainly because it's the **cause** of many of those diseases: diabetes; high blood pressure; arthritis; heart disease; a boatload of cancers; etc—which is when we **stopped** having a problem calling it a "disease."

So the only question left is: what disease are we talking about?

Well, it wasn't that long ago that no less a body than the American Medical Association, after a zippy 30 years of thinking about it, finally declared **obesity** to be a disease, and to let us know that we're smack-dab in the midst of an obesity **epidemic**!

And while we have only a minor problem with the "obesity epidemic" part—anyone with at least one good eye can see that that's what's going on in this country—we have a major problem with the first part: stating that "obesity" is the disease.

And why do we have a problem with that?

Because by calling the disease "obesity," that would seem to imply that, if you can just get rid of the **obesity**—through dieting, exercise, pills, etc.— you will have gotten rid of the **disease**, which is simply not true:

Look, right after World War I, no one went around saying, "We're in the midst of a worldwide **coughing** epidemic," even though that's what it looked like.

No, what they said was, "We're in the midst of a worldwide **flu** epidemic;" the coughing was just a **side effect** of the disease—a **symptom** of the disease—but it wasn't the disease—any more than wanting to eat, drink, and pee all the time **is** diabetes; or a runny nose **is** a cold; or swollen ankles **are** congestive heart failure.

No, all those things—the eating/drinking/peeing; the runny nose; the swollen ankles—those are all **side effects** of a disease—**symptoms** of a disease—but they're not the disease.

And so it is with obesity: obesity is not the disease; it's only a **side effect** of the disease—a **symptom** of the disease—but it's not the disease, and you don't cure a disease by getting rid of its side effects, no matter how good that might make you feel in the short run. You cure a disease by curing the disease. Period.

And, as it happens, once you cure the disease, any of the disease's side effects disappear all by themselves, without you having to give them a second thought, since there's nothing left to sustain them.

Look, if getting rid of a disease's side effects had any impact whatsoever on curing the disease, itself, we'd now be the **thinnest** nation on Earth, rather than one of the fattest, since, the last time I looked, all we've been doing, the last 50 years or so, is trying to get rid of that side effect—first with the Stillman Diet, then the Atkins Diet, then the Last Chance Diet, then the Beverly Hills Diet, then the Mayo Clinic Diet, then the Cambridge Diet, then the Scarsdale Diet, then the South Beach Diet, then the Zone Diet, then the Keto Diet, then…well, how much time have you got?

No, if getting rid of a disease's side effects—and who **hasn't** lost 20 or 30 pounds on one of those—if getting rid of those side effects had any impact whatsoever on curing the disease itself, we'd now be the **thinnest** nation on Earth, instead of one of the fattest.

Which proves, beyond a shadow of a doubt, that getting rid of a disease's side effects does absolutely nothing to get rid of the disease, itself.

Which is why, rather than giving you still one more way of getting rid of that side effect—in other words, giving you one more "diet," that, like all the ones that have come before it, will do nothing for you in the long run—we finally decided that **enough is enough** with things like that, and made it our job to go after something that **wouldn't** fail you: that would cure you of the **disease**, rather than just get rid of the **side effect** of the disease.

So, that's what we'll be doing here.

And please understand: we know exactly what the AMA was driving at when they decided to call "obesity" a disease: what they were talking about was a whole **spectrum** of things—mental and physical—that, **taken together**, lead to an excess accumulation of body fat—a.k.a., "obesity."

However, once again, the danger in doing that—and the reason we object to it so strongly—is that, by calling "obesity" the disease, you give the impression that, if you can just get rid of the **obesity**, you'll have gotten rid of the **disease**, which is like saying: if you can just get a lung-cancer victim to stop coughing—say, by giving him a gallon of Robitussin—you'll have cured him of his disease—which, of course, is total nonsense!

So, that's why we're so reluctant to call the disease "obesity."

Unfortunately, for a number of reasons—the AMA's announcement high among them—it happens to be more convenient to, in fact, refer to the disease as "obesity" (as we've done in this book's subtitle and elsewhere), even though it's not.

However, don't for a minute think that any extra body fat you might be carrying around is "the disease." It's not. Which means that simply getting rid of that extra fat won't be curing you of the disease, no matter how many "diet experts" try to convince you it will. It won't. Which is why we won't spend a minute of our time or yours going after that trivial side effect.

So, the question becomes: if "obesity" isn't the disease, what is?

And the answer to that is simple: the disease is: **abusive eating**: consuming more food in general—and more of certain foods in particular—than your body has any physical need for. In other words, eating for reasons **other** than "physical," no matter how "physical" they might feel.

Which is why we mentioned, early on, that, even though this country is, in fact, in the midst of an obesity epidemic, we actually have a problem **calling** it that.

Why?

Because, again, that would seem to imply that "obesity" is the disease, which it's not.

Which is why, instead of calling what's going on in this country an **obesity** epidemic, we'd prefer calling it what it really is: an **eating** epidemic, with the obesity being merely a trivial, though deadly, **side effect** of the epidemic—and, until you cure the disease that's **causing** the epidemic, you have no hope of **ending** the epidemic.

So, that's what we'll be doing here: helping you cure yourself of the disease of **abusive eating**, and, by doing so, eliminating all the **side effects** of that disease, the primary one being an excess accumulation of body fat—a. k. a., overweight and obesity.

Glossary

Addictive: The property of a substance that makes you want to consume it when you're not, and makes it impossible to **stop** consuming it once you start.
Adults: People able to exert some control over their own lives.
All-you-can-eat Restaurants: "Bottomless pits," where you feel obligated to eat 10 or 20 pounds of food because they let you.
Anxiety: Feeling of helplessness that arises when you lose control of your life situation.

Bathroom Scale: Instrument invented during the Spanish Inquisition to measure torture.
Body: Your constant companion
Body Fat: Nature's reminder that calories don't always vanish from the universe just because they vanish from sight.
Body Size: The size of your body
Bodysize: Formerly known as "fat" or "weight"; what abusive eaters lose when they turn themselves into normal eaters.
Burn-out (Muscle): Premature muscle "shutdown," due to trying too much too soon.

Calorie: A unit of heat-energy that fuels everything we do: thought, muscle function, food processing, body temperature maintenance, etc. When "number ingested" exceeds "number burned," excess is stored as body fat.
Champing at the Bit: What horses do when they're anxious to run.
Challenge: Asking more of something than it normally gives.
Control: Enforcing limits on your own or others' thoughts and actions.

Couch: Piece of household furniture designed for comfort
Couch Potato: Someone who spends inordinate amounts of time on a certain piece of household furniture.

Diet: What you eat.
"Diet:" A program that **changes** what you eat, for the purpose of helping you lose weight/bodysize.
Dream-world Slimming: Losing pounds per day, day after day; i.e., something that can only happen in your dreams (see also: **Real-world Slimming**).

Enemy: A non-friend: someone or something that is out to harm you or keep you from achieving a goal. Refers here to what your Subconscious Mind becomes when you try to "diet" your excess bodysize off.
Evolution: The horse we all rode in on.
Exercise: Method of getting fit and losing bodysize by **using** calories, rather than **restricting** them (see, for contrast, **"Diet."**)
Exercise Pushers: People who try to get you fit and trim by doing something **positive**—exercise—rather than something **negative**: starvation.

Fat: Chemical that evolution has chosen for our bodies to use, to store most of our excess energy.
Fitness: Measure of your ability to meet life's challenges, both physical and mental.
Fitwalk: What you go on, to get yourself fitter and to lose some bodysize.
Fitwalkers: People walking themselves fit.

Fitwalking: Walking as fast as you comfortably can for as long as you comfortably can.
Fitwalking Story: Exercised muscles pulling fat from storage to "recharge their batteries" and build themselves up.
Forbidden Fruit: Food whose consumption you can't really control and don't really want to.
Future: Something to look forward to or dread, depending on what you do each day to shape it.

Goal: The best way to bring order out of chaos.
"Gonzo:" Anything done to excess.

Habit: Anything you do automatically, day after day.

Infallible: What Mommies and Daddies are, till we become one.

Laws of Eating: The more you eat, the more you
>> want to eat
>> need to eat
>> can eat.
> The less you eat, the less you
>> want to eat
>> need to eat
>> can eat.

Life-expectancy Chart: A reminder that there's more to getting fit and losing bodysize than simply **looking** good!
Liposuction: A procedure where fat gets sucked off your body.
Liposuction Machine: A metal device, sitting in your surgeon's office, or the leg muscles you were born with.
Loophole: Something you can slip through when nobody's looking.

Losing Bodysize: Something done with great difficulty, by crushing your mind and body in a vise (see "Starvation Diet"), or with great ease, by turning yourself into a normal eater and walking as much as you possibly can.
Lottery: Game of chance which millions play but, statistically speaking, no one ever wins (see also **"Starvation Diet"**).

Metabolic Furnaces: Exercised muscles, which give excess calories the chance to be **burned**, rather than **stored**.
Money's-worth: What you should get from things that **enrich** your life, not **destroy** it.
"Murphy" Storehouses: Places where you really want your excess body to leave, so that's where it won't (see also: **Non-"Murphy" Storehouses**).
Murphy's Law (General): "If anything can go wrong, it will."
Murphy's Law of Bodysize Loss: "Wherever you really want the bodysize to leave, that's where it won't."
Muscle: Protein-rich body tissue where the majority of ingested calories are burned (see also: **Metabolic Furnaces**).

Non-"Murphy" Storehouses: Places where you don't care if they get emptied of their stored fat, so they do.

Politican: Someone who tells us what we want to hear (see also: **Tabloid**).

Real-world Slimming: Something that happens at the rate of an ounce or two per day (for contrast, see **Dream-world Slimming**.)

Shortfall: The difference between what you want or need and what you actually get.

Side Effect: The unavoidable consequence of trying to achieve a **primary** effect (lung cancer in smokers, cirrhosis of the liver in drinkers, etc.)

Slave: Someone whose life is being controlled by someone or something else.

Sore: An "ache-y" feeling in muscles, tendons, etc., due to those things being torn down but not yet rebuilt.

Starvation: Death due to lack of food.

Starvation Diet: Time-honored way to take off 20 pounds and put back 30!

Starvation Patrol: An imaginary group of people empowered to arrest Mommies who don't feed their children every 20 or 30 seconds.

Subconscious Mind: Portion of your brain designed to keep you alive and help you solve problems; receives most of its programming in infancy, therefore its "solutions" are often "infantile," and bear little relation to what would **really** solve the problem.

Tabloid: Newspaper, sold mainly in supermarkets, that tells us what we want to hear (see also: **Politician**).

Targets: Performance goals.